GO FOR GREAT!

DR. LIZ'S GUIDE TO THRIVE AT EVERY AGE

Dr. Liz Lyster, MD

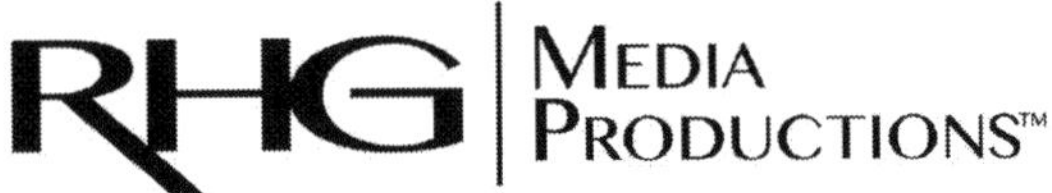

Published 2019
Printed in the United States of America

Print ISBN: 978-0-578-56848-5

RHG Media Productions
25495 Southwick Drive #103
Hayward, CA 94544

For Michael

TABLE OF CONTENTS

PRAISE FOR "GO FOR GREAT"

Dr. Liz Lyster's book **Go *for* GREAT: *Dr. Liz's Guide to Thrive at Every Age*** is an amazing combination of information, practical suggestions, real life stories, and useful knowledge you can take with you to your own doctor. She addresses the time of change in a woman's life, not only to educate women, but also their significant others. Not just a great source of information, this book is written in such a way that it is practical, easy to understand, and apply. I highly recommend **Go *for* GREAT** not only to any woman approaching "middle age" but also to those who love her and wish to understand what she's experiencing and to support her.

Elizabeth Clamon, Naturopath
www.ElizabethClamon.com

At last, a guide for midlife women written with an enjoyable, practical, and knowledgeable approach to safe and effective hormone replenishment. **Go *for* GREAT: *Dr. Liz's Guide to Thrive at Every Age*** is meant to empower each and every woman to participate fully in her self-care toward vital, healthy aging!

Patricia H. Baldwin, Nurse Practitioner,
Certified Menopause Practitioner
www.naturalhealthstyle.com

Do you want to feel your best AND do your best? Look no further than this book! In her powerful book, **Go *for* GREAT: *Dr. Liz's Guide to Thrive at Every Age***, Dr. Liz describes how, at any age, women and men can achieve optimal health-to truly thrive! When it comes to explaining the stages of our health as we age, separating the myths from the truths, and identifying specific tools to thrive, Dr. Liz has written an important guide that will be a valuable resource for all of us. Her vast expertise and wisdom are shared in a supportive, compassionate way and will be a consistent companion for those seeking to improve and maintain optimal health. Don't just focus on surviving, empower yourself and those you care about to truly thrive! Make the life-changing choice to **Go *for* GREAT** with your inspirational advisor, Dr. Liz, by your side!

Wendy K. Benson, MBA, OTR/L and Elizabeth A. Myers, RN
Co-Authors, *The Confident Patient*
2x2 Health: Private Health Concierge
www.2x2health.com

As I sat there and read Dr. Liz's book, I couldn't help but think of all of the changes that are currently going on inside of my body as I age, both good and bad. It is written with ease. A comprehensive, engaging dialogue. You can't help but to "get it." I felt like I was sitting right next to her in her office. I love the way she explains hormonal imbalance and treatment options for both myself and my husband. This is a must-have book on your reading list if the goal is wellness during "the change." Thank you, Dr. Liz

April Mahoney - Podcaster, Author, Poet
www.blogtalkradio.com/aprilmahoney

Want to feel young, energetic, and perform at your best? With sincerity and integrity, Dr. Liz clears out all the confusion, frustration, and scary myths around hormonal therapy. Awareness is always the first step of liberation. A must-read revelation book so you can thrive, say goodbye to unnecessary struggle, and enjoy great intimacy and ultimate harmony.

Naomi Bareket, Speaker, Author, Trainer
www.naomibareket.com

Dr. Liz cleared up so many misconceptions, myths, and just plain confusion about "the change." Knowledge we think we have adopted, but gets murky over the years, or is just plain wrong, was "dumbed down," regular-people speak, that I totally appreciated. This is information that can change not only the way women (or men), look at life but also the way they live their lives. Thanks, Dr. Liz, you are always entertaining, but this is simply up to date, vital information that's easy to read!

Renee Navarro, 58-year-old woman, wife, mom
www.melaleuca.com/reneenavarro

Dr. Liz's new book, ***Go for GREAT***, has a number of excellent aspects. I like how well-organized it is. Dr. Liz's stories about her patients are inspiring and easy to relate to. It is obvious that Dr. Liz is not only an expert but also a compassionate and reliable guide for her patients. I enjoy the depth and breadth of her book, without it being too much to digest. The author's vulnerability about her own story adds a warmth and personal touch that is a lovely background to the science and technology presented in her book. I believe that readers with questions about aging and hormonal health will find their answers in this informative guide.

Rosie Bank, Certified Integrative Nutrition Health Coach
www.rosiebank.com

This book is a must-have for any woman going into menopause or already in menopause. We've been led to believe that hormone replacement therapy will cause cancer—it doesn't! Dr. Liz Lyster breaks down the myths of hormone therapy that have left millions of women miserable and suffering from weight gain and brain fog. She gives you step-by-step guidance on how to get the support you need to make the right choice for you. Her book is refreshing, direct, and very readable. It will remove the fear that was getting in the way of you being your best self. As you read it, you'll begin to feel more relaxed and hopeful. If you are tired of feeling off, unwell, or "not your normal self," get this book and learn how to have vitality right now. You deserve it!

Kimi Avary, M.A., Relationship Navigation Specialist
www.ConsciousCouplesNetwork.com

In her latest publication, ***Go for GREAT: Dr. Liz's Guide to Thrive at Every Age***, Dr. Liz has presented her findings in the most comprehensive, reader friendly manner available in the current marketplace. From cover to cover, in a few hours, one can learn more regarding basic information and the role of individual common sense than by scouring a myriad of periodicals and scientific manuscripts. She combines facts and reality, opens the questioning mind, and provides a path for everyone to follow. The anecdotes and personal revelations make the content meaningful, believable, and approachable. You will feel you've made a friend who genuinely cares. I highly recommend this book as a stand-alone for the novice or well-informed, regardless of age or gender.

Susan Alpert, Author & Speaker
www.susanalpertconsulting.com

Dr. Liz Lyster's book ***Go for GREAT: Dr. Liz's Guide to Thrive at Every Age*** is a terrific handbook for every woman experiencing the trials and tribulations of menopause. There are so many misconceptions and fallacies regarding menopause and aging that a handbook that is easily read is a dream come true. I loved that Dr Lyster wrote her handbook as if she was having a conversation with the reader. So many questions that I didn't even realize I had were answered in a concise and unambiguous manner. All women will love to have this book by their bedside as a reliable reference whenever a question about aging and menopause occurs. Thank you, Dr. Liz for your creative handbook!

Susan Samueli, PhD – Co-founder Samueli Foundation
www.samueli.org

Dr. Liz's **GREAT** process cuts through so much misinformation. Her book gives a clear picture of what I need to do to feel good and live the life I want. The thriving section is motivational with tips that are doable in real life, which I find helpful and achievable. This book is an easy read that I refer to often whenever I need a pick-me-up during the day.

Denise Lynn McQueen Ms.T., Performance Coach
www.deniselynn.com

Dr. Liz beautifully demystifies hormonal therapy through providing plenty of facts, laying out benefits, and giving tools that assist us in truly 'Thriving at Every Age.' I wish this easy-to-read book had been available to me when I entered menopause, saving me from long stretches of low libido and energy.

Dr. Elsbeth Meuth, Bestselling Author of *Sexual Enlightenment*, Co-Founder of TantraNova Institute.
www.tantranova.com

In her engaging book, ***Go for* GREAT**, Dr. Liz Lyster demystifies essential matters characteristically associated with growing older. Through her narrative discussions and case studies, she presents vital solutions and pulls together the frequently misunderstood and mystifying pieces of the menopausal and hormonal puzzles. Dr. Liz's passion and expertise will undoubtedly inspire and encourage readers to become empowered stakeholders in their lives to improve and enrich their healthy aging journey. Every page provides insightful understanding and awareness of our bodies, how they are impacted by "the change," and reveals practical remedies and resourcefully effective Thriving Tools that can be implemented so we can all ultimately **Go For GREAT!**

Holley Kelley – Founder of Latter-Life Planning Institute, & Host of Aging GreatFULLy Show
www.HolleyKelley.com

ACKNOWLEDGMENTS

As with most births, a lot of support goes into the process of writing a book. Not in order of importance, I acknowledge the following people for their support: my husband, Michael, my number one fan and supporter in everything I do. Rebecca Hall Gruyter, my publisher for this and several other book projects–you were there for me every step of the way, and I thank you. Denise Lynn, you have been there for me for the last few major periods of my life, and I look forward to our friendship through the rest of our lives. My parents, Dr. Norah Gutrecht and Dr. Jose Gutrecht, who continue to love and support me through all of my endeavors. My kids, Anthony and Charlie, who continue to teach me and challenge me to become a better mom. Every person who has had a part in the successful making of this book, including Jamie Nease for the cover photography, and every person who supports me in improving my ability to get my message out, including Ed Tate, World Champion Speaker and Coach. Last for now, I acknowledge my patients in my practice, including many of my friends–you inspire me to keep going, to keep helping people one at a time to feel your best so you can do your best. You are the leading examples in my life that you don't have to "just" accept getting weaker or sicker as you get older; instead, we can Go for GREAT.

FOREWORD

The body of a woman, the child-bearer, is so miraculous and complex. Throughout a woman's life, there are so many changes that the body makes from becoming a woman in the teen years, through the child-bearing years, and, finally, into menopause.

However, as I was growing up (as a Baby Boomer), going to nursing school, bearing children, and going through "the change of life" (no one said "menopause" in polite company back then), one was never supposed to talk about these changes. Even doctors appeared as uncommunicative—and as clueless—about what was happening with our bodies as we were. This invaluable and indispensable book by Dr. Liz Lyster would have become the Bible for women like me as we rather blindly stepped into the phases of menopause. Unfortunately, this was not the case for me, but I am happy that it can be for you.

Hormones, like so many health topics, have been kept very much in the shadows as I have aged. The average person just knew that women could be "too emotional," even "hysterical," and no one knew what was truly happening or how to support us. When they called it "the change of life," they were not kidding. With two daughters and myself, my poor husband had all sorts of emotional women in his life. No wonder he spent so much of his time at work or on the golf course!

By the time I entered menopause, the woman I would have gone to with all my questions, my mom, was no longer with us, and I had no one else to talk to about it. When I did approach my doctor, I was given a lecture on hormone replacement therapy and the link to breast cancer, and I chose not to participate (until recently).

I really would have loved a doctor in my life like Dr. Liz, who truly understands what a woman's body needs and can explain it in terms a novice would understand. Instead, I felt very alone and isolated with no one and nowhere to turn for support.

Why is it that hormones are not studied in depth in medical school, nursing school, or clinical practices? When I look back on my nursing school experience, the topic of the endocrine system and the hormones they produce were only briefly explored in physiology and care for older adults. Even today, many doctors still don't have the training to help menopausal women with the symptoms that their changing hormones can cause, like hot flashes, insomnia, and, in numerous cases, sexual dysfunction—symptoms that for some can continue for fifteen years or longer.

Hormones are the key to an effective and efficient function of the body, which should be truly loved with vibrant aliveness. Yet balancing hormones seems to be a practice of last resort. I love the fact that it is not "hormone balance," as in once you attain it, you never have to do it again. The body is dynamic, and as such, the hormones need "balancing" on a continuous basis throughout life, especially as we reach menopause.

There are so many ads these days for male-enhancing drugs as the man grows older, but what about the interrelationship of all the hormones in the body? It is not just sex but living life to its fullest that is important as men age. I can honestly say that my relationship with my husband has continued to be rich and vibrant. He still continues to curl my toes.

In this book, Dr. Liz gives us a blueprint of our bodies and the hormone balancing that is necessary to be vital and energetic. She talks about how to take care of our bodies day-to-day to keep vibrant and to age gracefully. She arms us with information so we can advocate for ourselves and our health—and yes, about our sex lives and changing libido.

(Have you noticed how many drugs and services there are to help men's sexual performance, compared to those for women?) Dr. Liz gives us an easy and clear way to discuss our hormonal health challenges with our physicians.

Truly, this is a breakthrough book that shines a very bright light on a topic that remains a mystery for many of our healthcare providers. Because hormones were not a topic that was studied in detail when I was in nursing school, I would love strongly to encourage medical/nursing schools to enhance their curriculum around hormones and to require hormone education in the continuing education credits for the professions.

Women so deserve to have an experienced professional lead us through the maze of hormones and their interrelationship with each other. Dr. Liz tells women the truth about hormones and their bodies, busting myths and offering solid knowledge and advice throughout the book. Because we CAN handle the truth!

As she notes so beautifully, "I wish for you to have the most vibrant health possible, for as long as possible. It is not about staying young forever. But what good is extending our 'lifespan' if we don't lengthen our 'health span?'" There is such truth in these statements for all of us.

I loved this book, and my intention is to get it into the hands of as many healthcare professionals I know, as well as women who will benefit from reading it.

How about you?

Linda F. Patten, Leadership Trainer for Women Entrepreneurs and Changemakers
President &CEO, Dare2Lead With Linda
www.dare2leadwithlinda.com
linda@dare2leadwithlinda.com

IMPORTANT NOTE

The information presented in this book is not intended to serve as medical advice or as a substitute for medical advice. You should always consult with your physician before starting, stopping or changing any aspect of your medical treatment. The ideas and information in this book and any related materials are meant to be used with your good judgment and your sole responsibility, in consultation with the guidance and care of your physician.

INTRODUCTION

Getting older is a privilege; feeling old is optional.

They say if you fail to plan, you plan to fail.

Do you think this is true about getting older? I think YES.

We load up our lives with people, activities, and other stresses, both positive and negative. We get through the day, hoping to survive today so we can plop back in bed tonight, to get ready for another round tomorrow.

Most people go through life paying attention to their health only when things break down. In other words, most people go to the doctor *after* they have a health problem, not before.

However, I have a feeling this is not you. You are not "most people."

You are not on this planet to just survive through the day. You want more.

You want to THRIVE.

I'm going to give you an easy, five-step formula to help guide you to thrive at every age.

My patient, who I'll call Poppy, started out as a heckler. Seriously. She attended a talk I gave on hormonal balancing to help with weight loss, and she stood up and heckled me! I don't remember her question or what I said back to her, but somehow, the next thing I knew she was in my office for her menopausal symptoms. She was suffering from low energy, emotional outbursts (I already knew about those), night sweats disrupting her sleep, brain fog, sugar cravings and weight gain.

At her first appointment, I ordered a detailed set of blood tests, and I started her on some bioidentical estrogen and progesterone. Within the month her night sweats were gone, her sleep was better, and she was able to begin losing weight.

After six months, no one in the office recognized Poppy's pleasant demeanor. Our cranky heckler turned into a smiling, happy person, on the right track to feeling GREAT.

Every day in my practice, I help people go from the level of surviving up to the level of thriving. In each part of my five-step formula, you will also get tips for success so you can do more than just survive – you can thrive as you go along in life.

Why I am aiming this book at women? Don't men need to know about what is going on during and after "The Change"?

The answer, of course, is yes – men need to be aware of what is going on with the women they care about and work with. But, when I looked up what was already out there for men, I found many books for men about menopause. What was hilarious and eye-opening were the reviews, especially the ones written by women. Some of the reviews said, "Yes, read this to your husband!" (i.e. bought for husband, husband did not read it). Another review said, "It's written like a travel guide to a place he has never been to." Well, guess what, ladies? He has never been there and he never will.

There are zillions of books now for women about "the change" - perimenopause and menopause, and a few for men too. What I decided to do here is include some easy-to-use tools for the men in your life, so that they too are able to not just survive, but to thrive in their relationships with women going through this time of life.

This book is challenging to write, because no one likes any of the words involved!

Seriously.

No one likes any of these words:

- Hormones
- Menopause
- Perimenopause (most people do not even know what it is)
- Aging
- Older
- "Silver"
- Any other euphemism for aging or getting older!

But folks, here's the deal with "aging": if we are lucky, we get older.

Most people equate getting older with falling apart. I beg to differ.

I think that getting older means we have more life experience and more knowledge about how life really works, *and* we can have the strength of mind and body to get the most out of these years.

I love helping women feel better year after year. But,

my work as a doctor gets really fun when I get to care for a woman AND her partner (she usually comes to see me first, then he follows, but not always).

My patients, a couple whom I'll call Rose and Evan, are each in their second marriage. They have two teenage daughters together, and they each have older kids from previous marriages. They want to keep the "spark" in their relationship alive, including being in good moods with each other and having a great sex life.

It makes me so happy when I think about how many people are affected by Rose and Evan feeling better. It is so important for their daughters to have parents who are feeling GREAT so they can support the kids in doing their best.

With Rose, I have helped her get her metabolism working again, so she can have energy for her everyday activities and still have some left over for her husband, all while keeping her hormones in good shape so her hair and skin are great (this keeps her sense of self at its best).

With Evan, we looked at the same "hormone symphony" – thyroid, adrenal, sex hormones, and more – and after tuning up all the different parts of the symphony, now his music sounds great as well.

Dr. Pat Allen, one of my heroines, asserts that women need to FEEL good in order to DO good, and that men need to DO good in order to FEEL good. I agree.

But what happens for men when they do not feel good due to the "normal" hormone changes that happen with age? I consider it my job to help everyone have their internal hormone environment be its best so that *all of us* – both women and men – can feel well *and* do well.

MY OWN JOURNEY THROUGH "THE CHANGE"

I found out I was in menopause when I was forty-three years young. I was writing my first book on menopause and I figured I should check my levels.

My results showed I was in menopause. What a shock! Two years later, the difficult marriage I was in ended. I regrouped and started working on myself – body, mind and soul – so I could move forward in my life toward true health and happiness.

I moved with my boys from southern California up to northern California for a new job, and I also reentered the dating world. This process included starting my own practice, turning fifty, celebrating turning fifty by climbing Mt. Kilimanjaro in Africa, and then, at age fifty-two, meeting and marrying my current husband, the love of my life.

This process was joyful and rewarding, but also hard work! I want to take you behind the scenes of the process I followed then, and continue to follow now. A process to feel GREAT, not just for a short peak experience, but on an ongoing basis.

I am part of a generation of women going through "the change" while at the same time navigating never-seen-before life stressors. We have new technological constants, including cell phones, email, and the influence of social media.

Twenty-four seven connectivity is not how humans are designed. We are designed with rhythms, cycles that include down time, rest and sleep.

Even my mother admits that raising kids is harder now, in the age of cell phones and the Internet.

Most women my age observed our mothers as working women. Now we deal with the aftermath of the "you can have it all" legacy of the end of the 20th century. We sure "have it all": stress, overwhelming responsibilities, and difficulty putting ourselves high enough on our own to-do lists.

From the moment I had my first hot flash at the age of forty-three, I have been lucky to know that hormone therapy, done the right way, is safe and effective. I put on an estrogen patch and never looked back. Since then, I have tried almost every variation on the theme of hormone therapy, so I have personal experience with the options I present to my patients.

I was also lucky to be raised by women (my mother, grandmothers and aunts, all from Argentina) who understood and demonstrated the importance of self-care.

My *abuela* (grandmother) Zelmira lived to be ninety years old. She was active until her late 80's, visiting with friends, and keeping her love of music and dance alive. She was the oldest of five siblings. The youngest of those five siblings is my *tia* (aunt) Ines, who as of this writing is 83 years young and dances tango every Sunday in Buenos Aires.

Now *that's* my idea of getting older!

Want to join me?

WELCOME TO DR. LIZ'S GUIDE TO THRIVE!

This guide is unique because it will show you my five-step formula to feel GREAT and thrive at every age.

This guide is for YOU, whether you are a woman in this

phase of life, or a man who wants to learn what's really going on for women going through "the change".

As an important side note, although in this book I use heteronormative language, I am joyfully aware of the variety of gender identities and relationships that exist. I am privileged to care for couples of all gender combinations, as well as help with hormone balancing for individuals of varying gender identity.

I take your reading these words as a sign that you want to have a plan to live your best life for as long as possible, to feel your best, have your best brain function, and to have energy to do the activities you enjoy, so you can be there in body, mind and spirit for your loved ones.

In the chapters ahead, get ready to:

- Gain knowledge
- Realize the truth about hormones
- Explore your expectations
- Advocate for yourself

and...

- Thrive!

My message: do not settle for what most doctors say – that you are "just" getting older, that you "just" have to accept feeling tired, foggy, weaker, and so on.

We are not going to settle. We are going for GREAT.

CHAPTER 1
G IS FOR GAIN KNOWLEDGE

As the daughter of two doctors, I never really thought too hard about my path to becoming a doctor. I kind of ducked my head down and after finishing high school at age seventeen, went to college, medical school for four years, and residency in OB/GYN for yet another four years. I got married, had my kids, got divorced, dated, and remarried.

I went into menopause at the young age of forty-three (after the kids, before the divorce). Since menopause, I have gone through so many of the physical and mental changes I address with my patients. Add to all of this the dozens of classes and hundreds of hours in personal development courses, therapy, you name it, and the result is a considerable "body of knowledge".

However, as one of my heroines, Dr. Christiane Northrup, says:

"I have the body of knowledge, but you have the knowledge of your body."

YOU have to listen to your body, and I do not just mean eat chocolate because your body told you to (which actually might sometimes be good advice). When you know something is "off" in how you are feeling, do not let a doctor tell you "everything is fine" or that you are "just getting older".

Speaking of getting older, aging is itself a modern "problem".

Two hundred years ago, only about five percent of women reached age fifty. Now, at least half of women can expect to reach age eighty-five.

MEN: While men's life expectancy is not quite as high as women's, most men can still plan to live long enough for their testosterone levels to drop low enough to increase their risk of heart disease, prostate cancer, weight gain, and loss of muscle mass. Also, the "grumpy old man" stereotype is due to lack of testosterone.

When women do not have enough estrogen and testosterone, they can have less energy, motivation, and muscle mass, as well as lower sex drive and metabolism. They can experience weight gain and as a result have a negative self-image.

The bottom line is that older men and women can both be really cranky with each other. Marriages fall apart. Or, couples stay together but with a big loss of sexuality and sexual intimacy.

This kind of sexual health and intimacy struggle is not inevitable. It does not have to be this way. Further into this guide I will share more about what we can do about it.

First, let's take a look at some of our biology as we age.

THE BIOLOGY OF GETTING OLDER

In *Being Mortal*, Dr. Atul Gawande asked a medical specialist on aging "whether gerontologists have discerned any particular, reproducible pathway to aging." The specialist replied, "No, we just fall apart."[1]

I beg to differ.

There is in fact a very predictable pathway to aging, characterized by a set of patterns of hormone decline.

Most of our hormone levels peak around age twenty, an age when most illnesses are lowest and our energy level is highest. This is the time when young adults, like my son and his friends, can pull all-nighters and go out the next day and work or function normally.

This is also a peak age for fertility and parenthood. Again, the baby can keep you up all night and you can still somehow function the next day pretty well. However, I did not say this is an optimal age to actually raise children. I am only talking about biology.

The pattern of hormone decline starts in our twenties and people usually begin to show symptoms after age thirty. For men, testosterone levels peak by age thirty and decline by one to two percent every year thereafter. This affects mood, energy, sleep, muscle strength and metabolism. For women, by age thirty or thirty-five, progesterone levels start to go down. This affects mood, menstrual periods, sleep patterns, and fertility.

In our forties some hormone levels continue a steady decline in both men and women, including testosterone, growth hormone and DHEA. Other hormones, such as estrogen in women, begin to fluctuate. In perimenopause, which can be up to ten years or more before a woman actually stops having periods, estrogen levels can be low or high or simply out of balance with progesterone, resulting in bad moods, "short fuse", menstrual irregularity, disrupted sleep, cognitive problems, fatigue, and the list goes on.

Around the average age of fifty-one in the United States, women will transition into menopause. The menstrual period becomes very irregular, skipping a month or more, and hormone levels have huge ups and downs. I call this "the stock market phase".

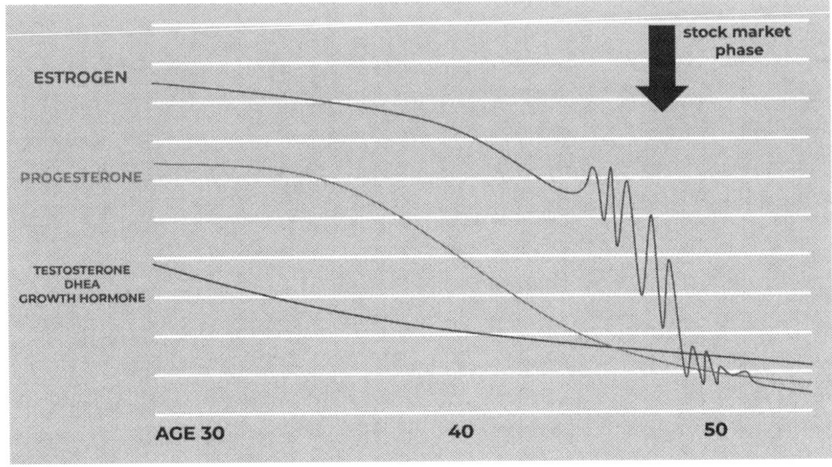

Figure 1. Patterns of hormone decline as we get older.

You can see how crazy the hormones can get.

Because people use the medical terms differently when they describe the stages women go through, let me present to you the three main stages. I am presenting them to you out of order to make it a little easier to understand "The Change".

THE THREE STAGES OF MENOPAUSE

1. PREMENOPAUSE = REGULAR PERIODS

"Pre-" (meaning before) menopause, describes a stretch of time from puberty to perimenopause (defined below). The premenopause phase starts when a young woman first gets her period and spans the years during which she has a regular monthly period. There might be some variation in her period due to stress, or long pauses such as pregnancy and post-partum, but overall her period is regular and she feels pretty "balanced".

2. MENOPAUSE = AFTER PERIODS STOP

A woman is officially in menopause when she has gone one entire year without her menstrual period.

When a woman who still has her menstrual cycle has her ovaries removed, this is called "surgical menopause". As you can imagine, this is usually a very abrupt ending of her cycle and ovarian hormone production. This situation has its own special needs.

I use the words "menopause" and "post-menopause" interchangeably. In other words, if you are "in menopause", it is also correct to say you are "menopausal" or "post-menopausal".

3. PERIMENOPAUSE = THE 10 OR MORE YEARS LEADING UP TO MENOPAUSE

Perimenopause refers to the years leading up to menopause. "Peri" means "around" as in a *perimeter* of a yard being the border around that space.

Unlike a perimeter, which you can clearly see and measure, perimenopause can go on for many years, as in ten or more years before a woman's periods finally completely stop. It is also not very clear to most women or their doctors when perimenopause actually begins. This is because symptoms of hormonal change can often either:

1. Not be clearly related to hormones, at least not according to classical teaching in medical school (such as sleep disruption or hair loss), or

2. Come and go, so there is no clear starting point to look back on.

Because of this, I like to use the word perimenopause very broadly, in order for people to recognize the hormonal aspect of health problems that many women start to have in their forties, sometimes as early as their thirties. I am referring to health issues like hot flashes and night sweats, sleep disruption, mood disturbance, depression and/or irritability for which women are usually given drugs to treat their symptoms, such as sleeping pills and anti-depressants.

I call these medications "Band-Aid® drugs", because they treat the symptom but not the underlying root cause of the problem, which is the hormonal imbalance that goes along with perimenopause.

In perimenopause, a woman might skip her period one month, or she might have a day or two of spotting instead of whatever is a normal period for her.

Does the spotting count as a period?

For the purpose of defining menopause, it usually *would* count. For example, if you go eleven months without a period then have a little bit of spotting, most doctors would consider you still in perimenopause and not yet officially in menopause.

NOT TO CONFUSE THINGS EVEN MORE: THE "MENOPAUSAL TRANSITION"

This is a term I use to describe the last part of perimenopause, in the last one or two years before a woman is completely done having her period.

This transitional stage is the hardest to define. As we said, in perimenopause, women can experience symptoms such as temperature fluctuation, mood and sleep disturbance, and irregular periods. I use the phrase "menopausal transition" when periods become even more irregular and further apart, usually accompanied by some or many of these other symptoms.

Some women sail through this transition with minimal discomfort or disruption of their lives, but as I always say, if this is the case for you, do not brag about it!

Can a healthy lifestyle and/or supplements help this transition? Absolutely.

As I will discuss in more detail in a later chapter, anything you can do to improve your hormonal and cellular environment will help you feel better during these life transition stages.

ISN'T THERE ANY CLEAR WAY TO TELL IF I AM GOING THROUGH "THE CHANGE"?

MENOPAUSE LAB TESTING – WHAT TO CHECK

Medicine is an art and a science. The definitions presented above are part of the "art" of menopause medicine. The science involved is helpful even if not terribly precise. Here are some tests we can do related to the phases of a normal menstrual cycle.

FSH

This is the main single blood test that doctors perform to tell if a woman is in menopause.

FSH stands for follicle stimulating hormone. FSH is released by the brain to stimulate the ovaries to function. The first half of a normal menstrual cycle is called the *follicular phase*. During this phase, FSH causes the ovary to grow and develop a dominant follicle, which contains what I call her "egg of the month".

In a woman having a regular cycle, FSH is at its lowest during her period. The first day of menstrual bleeding is called "Day 1" of the cycle. It is common to test the level of FSH on Day three of the cycle as a measure of fertility. The FSH level this early in the cycle should be low (less than 5) in the presence of good ovarian function, which also means better fertility.

As menopause approaches and ovarian function declines, the FSH level goes up (in most labs, this means a level over 25 or 30). An FSH level above 30, measured at least twice, more than six months apart, usually confirms menopause.

Why six months apart? Because in perimenopause, the FSH level can fluctuate. Look at the "stock market phase" where the hormone levels and symptoms can go up and down over weeks or months.

ESTROGEN

Estrogen is the main hormone of the first half of a menstrual cycle. When a woman's periods start getting irregular, and after menopause when the periods stop altogether, the ovaries can continue producing estrogen.

Estrogen is the main hormone responsible for female characteristics, such as:

- less hair on our face/bodies and more on top of our head
- softer, smoother skin
- higher voice
- female body contours
- breast development
- female fat distribution – hips and buttocks

Estrogen also

- improves mood/helps relieve depression
- stimulates and thickens the lining of the uterus (making a nice environment for a possible pregnancy)

The best time to check an estrogen level (usually the *estradiol* test) is on Day three of the cycle to check fertility (along with the FSH level). All other days of the cycle, the result must be interpreted as part of a whole panel of hormones. Eventually, the ovaries stop making any estrogen. Once a woman is in menopause, her estrogen level will usually be low.

Levels of estrogen typically start to get irregular when a woman is in her forties. Other factors can cause estrogen to fluctuate at any age. Unfortunately, when a woman suffers from mood problems related to fluctuating estrogen levels, she is usually given a "Band-Aid® medication" to treat her mood, instead of getting her hormones checked.

PROGESTERONE

Ovulation is in the middle of the cycle, during which the egg is released from the dominant follicle. As the egg floats away down the tube towards the uterus (and possibly towards uniting with a sperm resulting in a pregnancy), the follicle tissue left in the ovary organizes itself into a *corpus luteum*, which is a little producer of progesterone. This second half of the cycle is called the *luteal phase*. The main hormone level we measure during this phase is progesterone.

Progesterone is the main hormone of the second half of the menstrual cycle. When a woman's period is irregular, her ovaries are usually not producing enough progesterone.

This hormone balances estrogen, and does the following:

- calms the brain
- helps with sleep quality
- helps regulate blood sugar
- acts like a natural diuretic (counteracts bloating)

Progesterone also:

- helps relieve anxiety
- stabilizes the lining of the uterus so a woman's period will be on time and not too heavy

The best time to measure a progesterone level is on Day twenty-one of the cycle, if a woman is still having a regular period. If the cycle is already irregular or gone altogether, a progesterone level is a helpful indicator of whether a woman is still ovulating. Once a woman is in menopause, her progesterone level will typically be very low.

OTHER IMPORTANT HORMONES IN BOTH MEN AND WOMEN

TESTOSTERONE

Yes, both men and women have testosterone. While men reach much higher levels of testosterone in puberty, in both men and women this level steadily declines as we get older.

Testosterone helps women AND men with:

- muscle development
- weight management
- mood and sex-drive
- sexual function
- mental sharpness/clarity
- overall sense of well-being

	MEN	WOMEN
Where is T mostly made?	Testicles	Adrenal glands
"Normal range" in most labs	250 to 1100	2 to 42
Good level to have	At least 600 ***	Most women feel best above 60 ***

Figure 2. Testosterone comparison in women and men.

***There is a lot of discussion/controversy about what is the best level for both men and women.

Too much testosterone can cause: facial or body acne, excess facial or body hair growth, hair loss (more in men than in women), and, rarely, excess level of aggression. I say rarely because what you know about the "grumpy old man" is not from too much testosterone but rather from too little. It really takes a lot of testosterone, more than most doctors would prescribe, to make anyone overly aggressive.

The testosterone level can be measured anytime during a woman's cycle, and on any day in men.

Is your man a boiling frog?

Men in midlife and beyond and often find themselves in a position similar to the proverbial boiling frog. If you throw a frog into boiling water it will immediately jump right out and save itself. However, if you put a frog into room temperature water and bring that water very slowly to a boil it will not notice the onset of a dangerous situation.

Men's level of testosterone gradually declines at a rate of one to two percent each year starting around age thirty. Symptoms of low testosterone include fatigue, weight gain, mental fogginess, and irritability. While there is great concern in the general medical community about testosterone causing prostate cancer in men, it is clear that for the most part young men do not get prostate cancer and older men primarily do get prostate cancer, most often coinciding with low levels of testosterone.

In the antiaging medicine world, low testosterone is considered a risk factor for developing prostate cancer. I know this might sound counterintuitive, but there is considerable scientific evidence to support this theory.[2]

DHEA

This anti-inflammatory hormone is made by the adrenal glands in both men and women. We reach our highest levels of DHEA around age twenty-five, followed by a gradual decline. We also see lower levels of DHEA in the presence of stress, in which case the adrenals have to prioritize and focus on making more cortisol to keep us going.

DHEA helps with:

- mood
- libido/sex drive
- anti-inflammation

This hormone converts into estrogen and testosterone, so in excess it can also give the side effects mentioned above of testosterone (some facial hair or acne). The blood level of DHEA should be measured as the test for the active form "DHEA-sulfate", which is DHEA-S at most labs.

CORTISOL

This "stress hormone" made by the adrenal glands creates energy and helps regulate blood sugar. Under physiologic stress, or as I like to say, "life as we know it", the adrenals release more cortisol. After there has been enough stress for a long enough time, the adrenals become fatigued and the cortisol level drops.

Our adrenals mainly make cortisol during the night while we sleep, with highest levels occurring early in the morning when we wake up. The cortisol level then gradually falls throughout the day. Levels can be measured in blood as a fasting blood test in the morning or in saliva with kits that make it easy to measure it several times throughout the day to see how the adrenals are really doing.

Cortisol is a classic example of how conventional medical doctors only address something if there is a severe excess or deficiency. When it comes to adrenal fatigue, most people fall in between and cannot even persuade their doctors to check it.

All of these hormones contribute to our experience of life.

I could really go on all day about hormones. We cannot live without them.

As hormone levels decline in men and fluctuate in women, the way we feel and perform in life and in our relationships can really be impaired. Let's give you some tips for success to help you thrive as you continue gaining knowledge.

BAD NEWS MAKES BETTER NEWS THAN GOOD NEWS

First, I want to empower you with a critically important skill: how to debunk scary health headlines.

President Bill Clinton once said, "Bad news makes better news than good news."

This is absolutely true about hormone therapy.

When I was an OB/GYN resident in the early 1990's, we lamented that only one out of six menopausal women were on hormone replacement therapy.

When bad news came out in 2002 about hormone replacement therapy for women in menopause, this number plummeted even further.

Even now, all these years later, I hear from women, men, and even doctors who think that all hormone therapy is dangerous. Both lay and expert people fear that women will get breast cancer and men will get prostate cancer from hormone therapy.

In fact, the scientific data shows the opposite.

Yes, it is true! After reading this book, you are going to be more up-to-date than most doctors on the safety of hormone therapy and how it can be used to replenish declining hormones as we get older.

YOUR HEALTH HEADLINE DEBUNKING SKILL

The skill is to understand the difference between *relative risk* and *absolute risk.*

I took statistics courses *three times*, in college, in medical school, and in my master's degree program, which is way more than anyone should ever do. We are not going to get into technicalities. I just want to give you some examples to illustrate the point of relative risk vs. absolute risk, and show you how to use this knowledge, which you can apply to every medical headline you will read or hear about from now on.

Simple example:

According to the Centers for Disease Control, the chance of me as a pedestrian being hit by a car is about 1 in 4300.[3] If I walk outside in the neighborhood twice, I double this chance. Saying I "double" the chance, which sounds really scary, is the *relative* risk. Meanwhile, the *absolute* risk stays extremely small, as there is still a 99.95% chance that I will NOT be hit by a car.

Here is a simple health example:

Birth control pills have a known increased risk of causing blood clots in the body.[4]

The *relative risk* is that birth control pills double this risk. Double! That sounds bad, right? And it doubles again if you smoke.

However. The *absolute risk* of getting a blood clot in your body while taking birth control pills, if you are a woman who does not smoke, is about five out of ten thousand (the exact number varies by age).[5]

This means that statistically, 9,995 women can safely use

the birth control pills without getting a blood clot due to the pills.

Among women who smoke, the *double risk* means that ten out of ten thousand women using the birth control pill will get a blood clot. How many women who smoke can use the pill without it causing a blood clot? That's right: 9,990.

The *relative risk* – double – seems very scary, while the *absolute risk* remains extremely small.

Now let's take the number one example of a scary headline related to hormone therapy – the increased risk of breast cancer associated with hormone treatments. We are only talking about statistics and numbers here; the explanation of the hormones is coming up in a later chapter.

The Women's Health Initiative (WHI) Study, first released in 2002, showed an "increased risk of breast cancer with hormone therapy." In our next chapter we are going to get to the many flaws of this study.[6]

For now, what did the numbers for this "increased risk" show?

In one group, nine women out of ten thousand taking the placebo (sugar pill) developed breast cancer. In the group given estrogen/progestin hormone replacement, thirteen women out of ten thousand developed breast cancer.

Quiz time:

Q: How many additional women got breast cancer if they were given the hormones used in the WHI Study?

A: Four.

Four out of ten thousand. This is the *absolute risk*.

Four out of ten thousand is *less than one* additional woman getting breast cancer out of every thousand women in this study.

What came out in the media?

A *thirty percent increase* in breast cancer.

This was calculated by the extra four women adding up to a total of thirteen women out of ten thousand.

"Thirty percent increase" sounds so scary!

Again, I do not want us to get bogged down in the technicalities of statistical calculations. My only point here is to arm you with this one critical tool to debunk almost every scary health headline you will see.

Bad news makes better news than good news, right?

To prove this, let me now tell you something most people do not know, not even most doctors.

These findings from the WHI Study were published in 2002. Three years later, another finding was published that sadly has stayed almost a total secret: in the WHI Study, another group of women given only estrogen without the progestin had FEWER cases of breast cancer than in the women getting the placebo.

WHAT?!? That's right; the women getting only estrogen had LESS breast cancer and lived longer than the women who got no hormone replacement at all.

You would not buy a car without looking under the hood. Now that you understand the critical difference between relative risk and absolute risk, you will not just "buy" a scary health headline without taking a closer look.

So what do you do now that you have gained all this knowledge?

Can you safely replenish your hormones as they decline?

Luckily, the answer is YES! Read on for Step 2 of our five-step formula for feeling GREAT.

Patient Name: You!

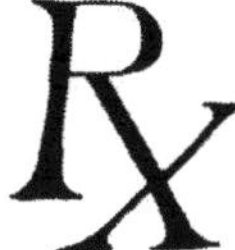

GAIN KNOWLEDGE

Tips for Success:

- Understand the major hormones that affect how you feel
- Ask your doctor for the right tests
- Pay attention to what is happening in your body
- Prepare for appointments with your doctor
- Debunk scary health headlines!

Signature: Dr. Liz, M.D.

CHAPTER 2
R IS FOR REALIZE THE TRUTH ABOUT HORMONES

People are afraid of the "H" word – hormones.

My passion is alleviating fear.

Did what you just learned in the last chapter start to calm down any fear you might have had about replenishing hormones that drop as we get older? I hope so.

It is not my goal to persuade you to use hormone therapy. It *is* my goal for you to not be afraid of using hormone replenishment to speed up the process of getting you back to feeling your best.

TOP THREE MYTHS ABOUT HORMONES AND MENOPAUSE

There are so many myths surrounding hormones, menopause and aging in general, that it is hard to know where to start to bust the myths and let the truth shine through. I have narrowed it down here to the top three myths I hear passed around as truth, even among doctors.

MYTH #1: "Hormone therapy is dangerous."

Truth: Effective hormone replenishment therapies exist that do NOT raise your risk of cancer or heart disease.

Those of you who have followed my writings know that I could talk for days to dispel this myth. In my medical practice, I see this myth causing the most suffering among women and men as they get older.

For women, the two hormones that go away after menopause are estrogen and progesterone. Replenishing them helps relieve most symptoms. Here are the two most basic points about hormone therapy for women, and one critical point for men, that will help you realize that there are safe hormone replenishment options during midlife and beyond.

1. Estrogen therapy is safest when used through the skin.

Whether it is vaginal estrogen to help with bladder function, comfort and response during sex, or estrogen applied to other skin areas to help symptoms like hot flashes and night sweats, what matters is to avoid using oral forms of estrogen. This is in order to avoid the cardiovascular side effects known to be increased with oral estrogen. Use a patch, gel, cream, suppository or subcutaneous pellet method instead.[7]

2. Progesterone is safest when it is *bioidentical.*

Whether it is a compounded progesterone product (cream or capsule) or a micronized progesterone from a regular pharmacy, your prescription must say the word "progesterone" on it. *Bioidentical* means it is the same form and structure as what your ovaries used to make before menopause. Bioidentical forms of hormones do NOT raise your risk of breast cancer, while the non-bioidentical forms, called progestins (an example of which is medroxyprogesterone) have been shown in multiple large studies to raise the risk of breast cancer.[8]

3. Testosterone does not cause prostate cancer in men.

If testosterone caused prostate cancer, we would see it more in young men, who have the highest levels of testosterone. Instead, we see a rise in the incidence of prostate cancer as men get older and their testosterone levels go down.[9]

The latest understanding of the relationship between testosterone and prostate cancer is the "saturation theory". This theory says that if prostate cancer is like a tree, giving it water will help it grow at first, but that if you add more and more testosterone, "the tree doesn't develop into a sequoia," as Dr. Tobias Kohler, Urologist and prostate cancer specialist says.[9] Removing testosterone helps at first in treating metastatic prostate cancer, but does not improve survival.

A huge 2015 meta-analysis of forty-two studies showed no statistically significant effect of testosterone treatment on the occurrence of prostate cancer. This is big news, but doctors are incredibly slow to change their practice based on scientific data.[10]

MYTH #2: "If I take hormones, I'll be stuck taking them forever."

Truth: Using hormone replenishment to relieve menopause-related symptoms does NOT commit you to using hormones forever.

The current position of the American College of Obstetricians and Gynecologists (ACOG) is that women having menopausal symptoms should only take and stay on hormone replacement therapy (HRT) for the duration of their symptoms.[11]

I do not agree with this statement.

I disagree with the ACOG position because of the many benefits of staying on HRT even after symptoms have been relieved.

For example, the amount of estrogen that helps a woman's bones stay strong is not enough to help any other menopause-related symptoms (like hot flashes or vaginal dryness). Therefore, if a woman no longer has menopause-related symptoms, her bones still benefit from a small amount of circulating estrogen.

I personally plan, and I comfortably recommend to other women, to stay on at least a tiny amount of estrogen forever, in order to avoid the devastating effects of a hip fracture. But just because I am super gung-ho about hormone replenishment does not mean you have to be.

Like I said before, I am not here to persuade you to use hormones, but I do want to alleviate the prevailing fear of hormones. If you have symptoms that are lowering your quality of life right now, please know that most women on HRT are able to stop taking hormones without getting their symptoms back again.

Luckily, the North American Menopause Society updated their position statement in 2017 in the form of a twenty-six page detailed document that states the following:

> "The concept of 'lowest dose for the shortest period of time' may be inadequate or even harmful for some women. A more fitting concept is 'appropriate dose, duration, regimen, and route of administration.'"[12]

MYTH #3: "I'm done with menopause."

Truth: Even after menopause-related symptoms go away, you are still "in menopause", and you might still benefit from some type of hormone replenishment.

Knowing the benefits of hormone replenishment is important for your long-term health. Even if you choose not to use systemic HRT, which circulates throughout your whole body and not just your vagina, a very small amount of estrogen can help your bones stay strong, or vaginal estrogen can keep your vagina and bladder tissue in good shape and help you avoid pain with sex or bladder infections.

While you will eventually be done having menopause-related symptoms, whether you use HRT or not, you will still be "in menopause". Some people use the term "post-menopause" to refer to this phase of life.

Nowadays, we all go online to research medical and health issues. Yet, the vast amount of information available can be hard to sort through at best, and terrifying at worst. After all, it seems as though one possible diagnosis for nearly any symptom is cancer.

I often say, "I've never seen anyone go on the Internet and feel better."

But I understand the predicament; you want to educate yourself and understand what is going on with your body. My challenge to you is to be aware of these myths so you can realize the truth about hormones.

WHY DOES IT MATTER TO KNOW THE TRUTH ABOUT HORMONES?

> "When women don't have enough testosterone, they don't like their husbands. When they don't have enough estrogen, they don't like anybody."

These are the humorous words of the late Dr. Bryant Herzog from Texas (so add a Southern drawl to the above quote).

We have already talked about the overall hormonal decline that affects us all as we get older. We have also looked at the "stock market phase" – the ups and downs that can last for years before a woman actually goes through "the change."

Our hormones are the chemistry of our emotions. They are our "internal weather." Just as you prepare for weather conditions outside, you can prepare for the emotional ups and downs related to hormonal fluctuations.

> OXYTOCIN is released by the brain during positive social interactions, during breastfeeding and during orgasm. It goes from the brain directly out to the body, improving mood, lowering blood pressure, and supporting blood flow through the skin and other tissues (this is what causes the skin to "glow" after having sex). It has a greater effect on women due to its interaction with estrogen.

Both men and women release oxytocin, also known as the bonding hormone. Oxytocin is one of the chemicals released when we feel attraction to another person. However, oxytocin works better in the presence of estrogen.

I call estrogen the "family glue."

Women in midlife experience ups and downs in estrogen levels, ending with an overall decline in estrogen. This usually coincides with children being older and getting ready to leave the home, or they have already left if one had kids at a younger age.

Less estrogen = less effect of oxytocin = less "family glue" = less bonding.

This new era of less hormonal bonding to the family leads to the time in a woman's life where she reconnects with her own dreams and goals and goes out into the world to achieve them. This requires adaptation on the part of both partners in a relationship. If she is single and looking to be in a relationship, she must realize she is trying to partner when her own internal hormonal environment makes it harder to do so.

By the way, if you or someone you know in midlife feels like leaving a relationship, please be aware of the big impact hormonal changes have on how we feel and the decisions we make. Seek to balance your hormones *before* making these kinds of life-altering decisions.

Men in midlife are also going through hormonal changes, as we discussed previously. For men, less testosterone means being less driven by the biological need for sex.

LET'S TALK ABOUT SEX

My patient, whom I will call Nell, age fifty-three, came to see me at a point where she could barely have sex with her husband due to pain and bleeding whenever they tried to have intercourse. Her husband, with her knowledge, was going elsewhere for sex. Their twenty-five year marriage was at stake.

Nell was very scared of using any hormone replenishment to help her feel good and get her body able to have sex comfortably again. We did not start her on systemic hormones, and instead had her start using only a vaginal estrogen cream. This brought elasticity and blood flow back to her vulva and vagina, so that within only a few weeks she was able to have sex without bleeding or terrible pain. Her marriage was completely back on track over the next few months, and improved even more when her husband came to my office as well.

Challenge #1 is being able to have sex comfortably. We talked about painful sex due to the loss of elasticity in vulvar and vaginal tissues from lack of estrogen. I always discuss this issue first with my patients who have low libido because it is normal to not want to do something that hurts.

Challenge #2: Low libido is another big challenge among the women I see in my office. Many women in midlife are missing the feeling of being "in the mood" for sex. Doctors may call this "hypoactive sexual desire disorder" but I stay away from these kinds of diagnostic labels (although I might use the codes to help my patients get their care covered on their medical insurance).

Lower hormone levels during perimenopause and menopause can negatively affect mood and sexual desire. In addition to estrogen enhancing the bonding action of oxytocin, it also helps lift up depressed mood. Put simply,

Estrogen helps depression and progesterone helps anxiety.

Progesterone, as we said earlier, calms the brain, which in addition to decreasing anxiety, helps improve the quality of sleep. By the way, here we can give another shout out to bioidentical progesterone, which is the only form that metabolizes in the way that results in a brain-calming effect.

It either needs to be micronized progesterone or made for you by a compounding pharmacy into a cream or a capsule. There are many forms of compounded progesterone, so do not give up if you need this brain-calming effect. The only side effect that can occur is feeling too sleepy the next day, in which case you can lower the dose or try a different form.

> This happened to me. The compounded progesterone helped my sleep greatly at first. Later, however, when my stress management improved and I was sleeping better with less of a cortisol surge during the night, I felt too sleepy the next day! My problem was solved using a micronized progesterone from my regular pharmacy.

DOES TESTOSTERONE HELP LIBIDO IN WOMEN?

After getting the vaginal tissues "rehabilitated" for comfortable and enjoyable sex, and getting the hormone levels in good shape, we can then address testosterone. In my experience, most women benefit from blood levels of testosterone that are above the reference ranges of most labs.

Having said that, raising your testosterone level usually does not help if you have:

- Other medications that lower libido (such as some anti-depressants)
- Disrupted sleep
- A partner who has impaired sexual function
- Resentment in your relationship

In a worst-case scenario, taking testosterone replenishment, can lead to a "libido mismatch" by making you have more sexual desire than what you or your partner can live with. In a best-case scenario, testosterone can boost libido, which benefits your motivation and drive in every area of your life, not just in the bedroom.

There are entire books on the topic of libido in women. Please see my Resources list in Appendix B. For our purposes here, I am commenting on the role of safely using hormones to help improve libido.

HOW ABOUT MEN?

Improving testosterone levels in men very often helps with energy, mood and sex drive. If a man has symptoms of low testosterone and his level is in the "normal range", his cellular receptors for testosterone may be resistant. In this case, some testosterone supplementation may still be of benefit. The best way to find out is to try supplementing and see if he feels better.

We have now seen how hormones are the chemistry of how we feel and interact with others. Now that you "Realize the Truth About Hormones," let's look at why this truth is not more widely known.

WHY DOESN'T MY DOCTOR KNOW THIS?

The pace at which information, especially bad news, gets out to the public is usually faster than the time doctors need to read about the studies, learn the science behind the data, and figure out what it means in practice.

It is actually worse than that. Even while new information emerges with the high speed of the Internet, new medical approaches can take decades to be applied in practice by doctors. One study showed an average delay of seventeen years between the publication of new scientific information in a medical journal and doctors actually using that information with their patients.[13] That is almost a whole generation!

I would say this is even true among doctors willing to try new approaches, which many are not. This is a case where the ego strength it takes to become a doctor can stand in the way of being a really good doctor, one who uses the latest information to benefit their patients. The ego can get in the way because new information challenges "the way we have always done things." No one likes change.

Another phenomenon we see now is the super-specialization of doctors. Endocrinologists, who are experts on the hormone-producing organs of the body and their diseases (including thyroid, pancreas, and adrenals), usually will not treat one patient's entire endocrine (hormone) system. For example, if a patient has severe diabetes, the endocrinologist will specialize in this and will not deal with their hypothyroidism.

Another problem, at least in American medicine, is that doctors often only treat extremes of illness. If they determine that your levels are "in the normal range", even if they are barely inside that range, then you are sent out the door, with your symptoms and your suffering unaddressed. We will address this again in a later chapter.

This breaks my heart. It also makes me mad.

WHY DOESN'T MY DOCTOR DO THE EVALUATION I NEED?

Every time I hear a patient say "You're the first doctor who has really listened to me," it makes me happy but it also makes me cringe. What is the matter with doctors? I know they mostly go into medicine wanting to help people. In practice, most of them end up too short on time to really be able to listen to their patients and help.

Being short on time with a patient is one factor that drives the Western medical approach of looking for the symptom that can be treated with a drug, in order to get the patient out the door.

You have to be "the tail that wags the dog." We will talk about this more in Chapter 4.

WATCH OUT FOR "DR. GOOGLE"

There is a popular meme that says, "Don't confuse your Google search with my medical degree."

While I think apps and other computer-assisted methods will improve health care going forward, one Harvard study showed that actual doctors did better than an app at coming up with a correct diagnosis when given the same information.[14]

As I like to say, I have never seen anyone go on the Internet and feel better.

I remember when patients first really started using the Internet to search for information. I remember some of my colleagues getting bent out of shape about the time it took to talk with patients about what they were learning on the Internet. These doctors felt personally disrespected by people going outside of their doctor-patient relationship for answers to their questions.

I realized that online searching was here to stay as a method for people to find information and answers about their health and their symptoms. Doctors cannot play ostrich by burying their heads in the sand and ignoring the fact that patients now have tremendous access to information through the internet.

There is a movement afoot in medicine today to be "evidence-based", which means it is important to evaluate studies carefully for their design, so you can then assess the quality of the results of the study. However, even in studies with a good design, there are still many pitfalls for all types of studies.

- Who funds the study? The maker of the drug, a university, the government?

- Who was included in the study as participants? Can the results be generalized to men and women, to kids, to all ethnic groups?

So far, our deep dive into learning about hormones, and the fact that scientific study results can be presented in misleading ways, shows us how much there is to learn and to watch out for when we read health information.

Now that you have gained knowledge and you realize the truth about hormones and hormone replenishment options, you do not have to be afraid. You can confidently use the right kinds of hormones to help you feel GREAT.

Let's go on to Step 3 of our formula.

Patient Name: You!

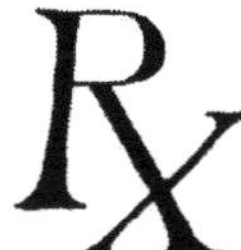

REALIZE THE TRUTH ABOUT HORMONES

Tips for Success:

- Some hormone replenishment options are safer than others
- Find a knowledgeable doctor who will check your hormone levels and take time to discuss your options
- Watch out for "Dr. Google!"
- Women: use estrogen through the skin (does not go to your liver first); use only bioidentical progesterone
- Men: use testosterone as neded to feel your best, under the right medical supervision

Signature: Dr. Liz, M.D.

CHAPTER 3
E IS FOR EXPLORE YOUR EXPECTATIONS

"HOW SOON WILL I FEEL BETTER, DOC?"

My patient Bonnie, age sixty-four, had been taken off her hormone replenishment regimen by another doctor. She was very busy with her work, babysitting her three little granddaughters, and her hobbies, and she was anxious to get back to feeling her usual energy and stamina. She was also in a new relationship with a great guy, and she wanted to actually feel good with him instead of "faking it." I told Bonnie what I tell everyone, which is that most people I work with feel better by the one month mark. Bonnie was not in this majority, and she was in a panic! About two months after starting her full hormone replenishment regimen, she was back to feeling fantastic again, and was sleeping well, thinking clearly, having a great intimate life with her partner, and even lost sixteen pounds.

We live in a fast-paced, fast-food, "get it now" mentality world. In my office, this translates into people wanting to feel better right now.

We all want a quick fix, preferably in the form of a pill to make our health issues instantly disappear. Modern medicine seems to promise this to us all.

This "quick fix" mindset makes it challenging to manage people's expectations.

I have good news and not-so-good news.

The good news is: You can feel better pretty quickly with hormone replenishment.

The not-so-good news is that "pretty quickly" can mean anywhere from a few days up to a few weeks, and at this point in medicine, I cannot say at the outset which group you will fall into. Eventually, I think we will be able to check your genes and predict whether you will respond to a particular medical treatment, and how quickly.

More good news: Most of the patients I work with feel better within a month of starting any kind of hormone replenishment. By "most" I mean about ninety-five percent of my patients.

"Better" can range anywhere from feeling a lot better to at least feeling like things are headed in the right direction. I see people back in the office after four to six weeks for the first follow-up appointment. I do this first follow-up so soon because I want to make sure my patient is in the ninety-five percent who are going in a good direction. If he or she is in the five percent, we review the plan in detail and make adjustments to get things on track.

After all, we are dealing with the human body.

Your body may be like a machine, but your hormones are more like a symphony. You have to work on all the sections of the symphony at the same time, including the strings, the percussion, the wind instruments, and so on. If any section of the symphony is off, the whole sound will be out of tune.

HORMONE TIME FRAME

Another factor in managing your expectations is what I call the "hormone time frame." It takes about eight to ten weeks until your cells fully realize that they are "under new management."

This is based on two sources. The first is based on the research of Dr. Bruce Lipton, author of *The Biology of Belief*, and the second is from my clinical experience over my career.

Dr. Lipton conducted research in cell biology.[15] My summary of what he discovered is this: if you take the nucleus (the cell's "brain") out of a cell, the internal processes (such as metabolizing and making proteins) of that cell will keep working for about eight to ten weeks. At that point the cell will die if it is not given fresh "instructions."

This time frame for cells to respond to new instructions goes along with my clinical experience with patients. Especially when a patient feels improvement with a particular hormone or supplement, if she stops using it, she will usually continue feeling okay for a few weeks, but after three months or so she will begin to feel the symptoms we sought to address, such as fatigue, brain fog, and so on.

MINDSET FOR HORMONE BALANCING SUCCESS

You get my point: hormone balancing is not a "quick fix."

Instead, it is an ongoing process that takes weeks at first, then continued close monitoring and adjusting for at least the first year. Eventually, you will get into what I call the "cruise-control" mode.

By the time a patient reaches "cruise-control" mode, they will have a good idea of how their symptoms respond to which hormones or supplements. This is why it is essential to be tuned in to your body and work with a responsive doctor.

In fact, taking care of your one precious body is a lifetime project.

Expecting to feel better and to stay that way forever is like going to the dentist once and expecting your teeth to stay clean and polished. Even with daily cleaning of your teeth, you still need to stay in the regular care of a dentist to keep an eye on things.

WILL HORMONES ALONE FIX HOW I'M FEELING?

Short answer: NO!

When I was practicing gynecology, I felt like a plumber. Women wanted me to go in and fix their female problems. These women were less interested in looking at their own role in their recovery and prevention of more trouble in the future.

Now I feel like a chemist. People want that "magic pill" or the one magic hormone potion that will bring everything into balance and make them feel great, without them doing anything else on their end.

Your role is as crucial as your doctor's, maybe even more important for your long-term hormone balancing success.

YOUR *PART* IN THE DOCTOR-PATIENT *PARTNERSHIP*

For you to have appropriate expectations of how you will respond to hormone balancing, we have to touch on some other key points.

In addition to the medical side of hormone balancing, i.e. the actual hormones being prescribed, there are three major areas that you have to address:

- Nutrition
- Exercise
- Spirit

NUTRITION

In my career, I am constantly approached about new diets and products to support weight loss. I have seen many approaches come and go over the years.

I think the food pyramid as we learned it in the past is wrong. We are designed to eat more lean proteins, more fruits, vegetables, nuts and berries, and fewer processed grains. As we get older, hormonal decline affects our immune system, women more than men it seems, resulting in food sensitivities that we did not have before.

As far as I am concerned, you do not have to become vegan, but you probably have some room to improve what you eat to support good hormone balancing.

EXERCISE

Sometimes I call this “the E word”, especially when people are not naturally drawn to exercise and do not particularly enjoy it. I like to substitute in the phrase “move your body.”

For those who do not get that nice mood boost from exercise, there is something called N.E.A.T. - non-exercise activity thermogenesis. This includes tips you have probably heard before: park further away, take the stairs instead of the elevator, sit with good posture (yes, this burns more calories).

> On the other hand, I recently saw a new patient, whom I will call Emily, who loves to exercise.
>
> Emily likes to do tough workouts at least five times per week, more if her work schedule allows it. She works out with two different trainers at her gym, and gets a huge stress relieving effect from exercise.
>
> With Emily, I have the difficult task of persuading her that the body needs time off the day after a hard workout in order to hormonally process the energy burning and growth hormone production that happens after exercise. It is equally hard to persuade her that activities that promote circulation, such as massage or yoga, are just as important for her cell environment, even for weight loss.

Among other nutrition and fitness gurus, I like the work of Haylie Pomroy, originator of the Fast Metabolism Diet. Her work emphasizes *variety* and *rotation* of different types of exercise, or moving your body. I am also impressed by Dr. Susan Pierce Thompson, the creator of Bright Line Eating. For links and more information, please see the Resources section at the end.

SPIRIT

In addition to the work of Dr. Bruce Lipton on the power of our minds over our bodies, I love and have followed for many years the work of Dr. Christiane Northrup. After writing many detailed and in-depth books about menopause, she now focuses on the power of our thoughts on our health.

By spirit, I include your mental state, your emotional health, your happiness in your life, and your relationship to "Source", whether you call that "God" or nature or any other name.

Dr. Northrup summarizes the power of our mind/spirit so well:

> "Thoughts are an important part of our body's wisdom because we have the ability to change our minds (and our thoughts) as we learn to grow. A thought held long enough and repeated enough becomes a belief. The belief then becomes biology. By choosing to move forward into health and joy, we can uncover the deep programming of our bodies and change it to support health."[16]

YOUNG FOREVER?

To finish up this step about exploring and managing your expectations, let's look at some mindset myths about aging in general.

Jane Fonda is another one of my heroines. Some of her latest work includes talking about "Life's Third Act," including an awesome TED talk by this title.[17] A quintessential celebrity representative of the baby-boomer generation, Fonda starts out the way I often do, by pointing out how much longer our life expectancy is compared to people three generations ago – thirty-four years longer on average.

This creates a modern problem, or as Jane Fonda prefers to say, a modern challenge. We have an opportunity to experience up to an entire third of our lives as a time to reinvent ourselves, as opposed to falling into decline. This requires our entire society to reimagine this "Third Act".

Each of us as we get older must re-examine our own level of health and function.

We do not have to function like people in their twenties. When we were in our twenties, we could usually pull all-nighters and not eat great and continue to function and manage our weight with relative ease. This is not the case in our forties, fifties, sixties, and so on. That is okay, because as I always say, there is a reason we do not want twenty-year-old's running the world.

In a youth-worshipping American society, we not only have to improve the care we take of ourselves and our health, but we also have to persistently challenge our society's view of "older" people.

MINDSET MYTHS ABOUT GETTING OLDER

To do this, we have to ask ourselves, "What societal beliefs have I unconsciously bought into?"

Have you bought into any of the following mindset myths (even a little)?

1. People are less sexual as they get older
2. People automatically decline as they get older
3. People get sick as they get older

Let's take these one by one, and look at the steps we can take in each area to heal ourselves from these beliefs:

MYTH #1: People become less sexual as they get older.

What I am talking about here is the mental shift and the mental personal work it takes to stay feeling sexy and to be sexual as we get older.

My primary expertise is in the physical caretaking, and the adjustments we have to make as we get older, in order to stay in sexual working order. This is an ongoing journey, and I am right there with you on this journey!

Speaking as a medical professional, it is often not easy for a patient to discuss sexual function with a doctor. In fact, many studies confirm how seldom patients bring up issues of sexuality, and emphasize that doctors have to be the ones to "break the ice" on this sensitive and possibly embarrassing topic.

It is also not that easy to talk about sexuality in an intimate relationship. When we are young, we do not have to; everything is in working order!

As we get older, life becomes busy and stressful, and sexual desire often decreases as sleep and mood disturbances increase. In addition to these mental changes, physical changes that occur as we get older can include less hormonal effect on, and less blood flow to, the genital tissues, resulting in more difficulty with erectile function in men and sexual response and orgasm in women.

Actually, it is not that easy to discuss matters of sexuality at all, and it is worse still in the relatively prudish American society. I have my OB/GYN profession combined with my personal South American family background to thank for my willingness to have these conversations with patients, as well as in my own marriage. I focus on the end goal – a satisfying and fulfilling intimate relationship, as defined by each individual person or couple.

2. MYTH: We inevitably decline as we get older.

Baby Boomer celebrities are doing their part to dispel this myth.

We as individuals all have to work on this. Hopefully we continue healthy eating and exercise habits from when we were younger, but most of us also have to eat and exercise differently.

I always say, "As the building gets older, it needs more maintenance."

What I mean by this is that decline is not inevitable, but it does happen for specific reasons. For example, many people treat their older body the same way they did twenty years before. This is not reasonable. You would not run your twenty-year-old car the same way you did when it was brand new. You would be more attentive to fixing problems as they came up and more on top of regular maintenance. This is exactly what we have to do with our bodies as we get older!

Many people also assume that mental decline with age is inevitable. The more we learn about brain science, the more we learn what we can do to preserve mental sharpness.

For example, research shows that standing instead of sitting improves blood flow to the brain and promotes core body strength and balance. Core strength prevents frailty, and balance helps prevent falling.

Hormones that help mental sharpness include thyroid hormone, estrogen and testosterone.[18]

Again, even though many people experience a slower mental process compared to when we were in our twenties or thirties, it is appropriate to repeat here that there is a reason we do not want people at those younger ages running the world. "Slower" mental processing can also mean a more reasoned and methodical response to the pressing challenges our world faces today.

3. MYTH: People always get sick as they get older.

My mom once observed, "I can't stand one more person retiring, then getting really sick!" It is true that many illnesses occur in the environment of lower hormone levels later in life, such as breast or prostate cancer, osteoporosis, and hip or spine fractures.

Also, in the presence of lower hormone levels, our immune system does not function as optimally, so we heal more slowly.

I remember when my son was twelve years old, and he was playing at a friend's house when a baseball hit his hand really hard. The next day, his thumb looked like a purple sausage. I took him for an X-ray of his hand (and if you know doctors, you know this is a big deal for me to be that concerned; usually we do not get too excited unless there is spurting blood or bones sticking out). The X-ray did not show a fracture, and within two weeks his hand looked completely normal. There was no swelling or bruising that remained, no pain whatsoever, and his hand was fully functional.

That is the speed of healing when we are young; this does slow down when we are older, and we have to respect this. If we do not honor the recovery process after illness or injury, we will just prolong it, or even make it permanent.

Also, if we do need surgery in our forties, fifties, sixties, and so on, we are better off if we go into it in the best possible overall health, at a healthy weight, with decent nutrition and decent mobility. It is never too late to improve our health.

MANAGING YOUR EXPECTATIONS

Now that you have explored your expectations, let me give you some tips to get really good at managing them as you work on this lifelong project called Going for GREAT.

As human beings we want results now. If I had a magic wand I would give everyone the gift of feeling great right this minute, and it would last forever.

But alas, we are human beings, who have to learn as we grow to look at the long game. It's a marathon, not a sprint.

Many people say life is short, but it is also long. As my 85 years old friend used to say,

"If I had known I was going to live so long, I would have taken better care of myself!"

BABY STEPS FOR LIFESTYLE CHANGE

We do not have to change every aspect of our lives or make many changes all at once. Small incremental changes are not sexy but they add up to better long-term health and wellness.

Proven steps to improve your "health-span":

- Do not smoke.
- Eat less.
- Move more. (between "work-outs")
- Connect socially – in person!

Each of these can be broken down into its own baby steps.

Reducing smoking lowers your risk of cardiovascular disease proportionally. That is, the fewer cigarettes you smoke, the lower your risk. Quitting is optimal, and of course lowers your cardiovascular risk the most. Lung cancer risk however, does not decrease until after you quit completely.

Eating less means going back to the days before "super-sizing." Even if you do not eat fast food, not to mention "super-size" fast food portions, did you know that in the 1950's the average size dinner plate was nine inches in diameter, compared to today's average dinner plate, which is twelve inches across? Correlated with these bigger plates are bigger servings of food: over the past fifty years, Americans have made the transition to eating more than twenty percent more calories per day, on average.[19]

I remember when I was a kid, the "small" size cup at a restaurant was eight ounces, which is what we use now as a water cup. The "small" size now is usually at least twelve if not sixteen ounces.

We already mentioned moving more. Park further away, take the stairs. It is true that these small steps make a difference long-term.

I can also add here another comment about moving *differently*. We mentioned that it is good to vary the type of exercise you do. Doing the kind of exercise called "burst" or

"Tabata" or "H.I.I.T." (high intensity interval training) can give you a short workout that burns more fuel than the type of workout that does not have variable intensity, like jogging at a steady pace on a treadmill. This is exactly the way stop and go city driving burns more fuel, whereas highway driving involves moving at a steady rate for longer stretches and burns less fuel.

This kind of burst exercise session is also good for you hormonally, in particular by increasing your body's production of growth hormone (GH). GH helps kids grow, but when we are done growing it continues to help with tissue and cellular repair. We make growth hormone at night while we sleep, so you absolutely must guard and protect your sleep quality.

The last of these small steps you can take towards feeling GREAT, is the importance of social connection. Scientific data continues to pour in about the health impact of social connection, including:

- Stronger immune function
- Less anxiety and depression
- Lower mortality

Lack of social connection may be worse for your health than high blood pressure or even smoking. Brené Brown says that when our human need for social connectedness is not met, "We don't function as we were meant to. We break. We fall apart. We numb. We ache. We hurt others. We get sick."

TRACK HOW YOU ARE FEELING

There's an app for that.

Really, there are a growing number of apps to help you track how you are feeling. Do you not like to use your smart device to track how you are feeling? Good old-fashioned pen and paper is fine too. I even have a chart I still give my patients that is a grid of one whole year on one page. There still is not an app that tracks symptoms and generates a one-page report for me to see patterns over several months.

In addition to the proven benefits of writing regularly in a journal, it is amazing how quickly people forget how bad they felt in the past. Our minds are helpful to us in this way; they often do not hold on to the negative details of how we felt before we got help.

I see this all the time in my practice.

Amelia told me at her first follow-up appointment six weeks after we started her hormone balancing program, that she only felt that her hot flashes and night sweats had improved. Luckily, before her initial visit, I had asked her to fill out a detailed history questionnaire and we had done a phone consultation to talk about how she was feeling.

At her first follow-up appointment, I reviewed several other symptoms we had initially discussed.

Hot flashes and night sweats? Better.

But also...

Brain fog? Better.

Sleep? Much better.

Pain with sex? Getting better.

Short temper with her kids? Better!

Bottom line? Track your symptoms. At first, it will be helpful so you can see what is getting better and what needs more adjusting. Later it will still be just as important, because we are not talking about hormone *balance*, we are talking about hormone *balancing*, an ongoing lifelong process.

STAY IN COMMUNICATION WITH YOUR DOCTOR

Find out from your doctor's office the best way to stay in communication.

Most doctors now have a way for you to email questions to them. Short, bullet-pointed questions are best for this format because this allows your doctor to answer more promptly. Sometimes your questions may require a short phone call.

If you have side effects, your doctor wants to know. If you stop taking a prescribed medication or a recommended supplement, your doctor needs to know.

I have a framed poster on my wall that says, "If all else fails, follow the instructions."

This might sound obvious, but you would be amazed at how often patients change the program we agree on, and then are surprised or unhappy that they do not get the expected results.

It is not about the doctor/person with authority telling the patient what to do. Remember Dr. Christiane Northrup's quote? "I have the body of knowledge, but you have the knowledge of your body."

Everything you feel, whether good or bad, is relevant to your successful process of Going for GREAT. Now you have gained knowledge, realized the truth about hormones, and you have explored your expectations so you can learn how to manage them.

We're ready for Step 4 of our formula.

Patient Name: You!

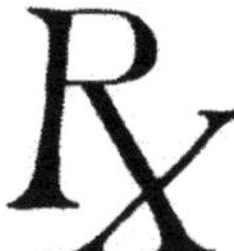

EXPLORE YOUR EXPECTATIONS

Tips for Success:

- **Life is long (hopefully) - treat it as a marathon, not a sprint**
- **Hormone balancing is an ongoing process**
- **Do your *part* in the *part*-nership with your doctor**
- **Baby steps may not be sexy but they count!**
- **Stay in communication with your doctor**

Signature: Dr. Liz, M.D.

CHAPTER 4

A IS FOR ADVOCATE FOR YOURSELF

As we go through life, we have a choice between two paths: one option is to "muddle through" as best we can, accepting the level of health we are lucky enough to experience.

The other option is to be proactive about our health. Part of being proactive is advocating for yourself.

BE THE TAIL THAT WAGS THE DOG

> My patient Anna came to me at age thirty-nine. She and her husband had been trying to get pregnant, and their efforts were not working. She was on thyroid medication. She was told her thyroid tests were "normal". We took a deeper look, both at the labs results being called normal, and also the thyroid medication she was prescribed.
>
> The conventional medical world has very standard, often limited ways of treating many conditions, especially low thyroid. There are actually many ways to treat hypo- (low) thyroid conditions. We made some adjustments to the type of thyroid medicine she was taking. Soon after, Anna got pregnant and gave birth to a healthy baby boy.

Most of the patients I take care of have been told at one point or another by a friend, loved one, or even a doctor, that they "just" have to accept feeling more tired as they get older.

If I could ban one word from the English language, it would be this 4-letter word: "JUST."

Maybe I can start by banning it from doctors' discussions with their patients. I have so many patients who were told by their doctor that they "just" have to accept that they are getting older, meaning there is nothing they can do to feel great energy, or have vitality and stamina.

Not true! There is so much more knowledge out there than what conventional medical care tells you to help you feel great at every age.

When I speak to people, I illustrate the range of doctors that exists in the world by standing with my arms outstretched. Along my right arm is "conventional medicine." This side of the spectrum is driven by disease management, symptom control with pharmaceutical drugs, and protocols developed in and applied to groups of people, not individuals.

On the opposite side of the spectrum, along my left arm, is "anti-aging medicine." This area of medicine is also known as regenerative medicine. At the extreme end of this side of the spectrum are the doctors who take care of the movie stars, doing every experimental treatment around the world that has any chance of helping someone recover from an illness or feel better. These approaches include treatments that are not accepted (or might even be outright rejected) by the conventional medical community.

I practice on the regenerative medicine side of this spectrum, but not at the extreme end. This side of the continuum emphasizes wellness, disease prevention by lifestyle, and using as natural of an approach as possible to achieve optimal health.

GET THE RIGHT TESTING

An example of advocating for yourself is in the area of testing. If your doctor is willing to do some testing for you (i.e. go beyond telling you you're *just* getting older and you *just* have to accept it), remember to go for better than your results being barely inside the "normal range."

This is incredibly common for men regarding checking testosterone levels. I have heard terrible stories where the doctor will not even check the level, even though the man is having many of the symptoms of low testosterone, including fatigue, brain fog, irritability, weight gain or decreased muscle strength.

One young man in his thirties was told that because he was still having erections, he could not possibly have a low testosterone level. Not surprisingly to me, this turned out to not be true; his level was nearly at the bottom of the range, exactly as shown in this cartoon (which I have framed in my office).

CONGRATULATIONS!
YOUR RESULTS ARE IN THE NORMAL RANGE
LOW
NORMAL
HIGH

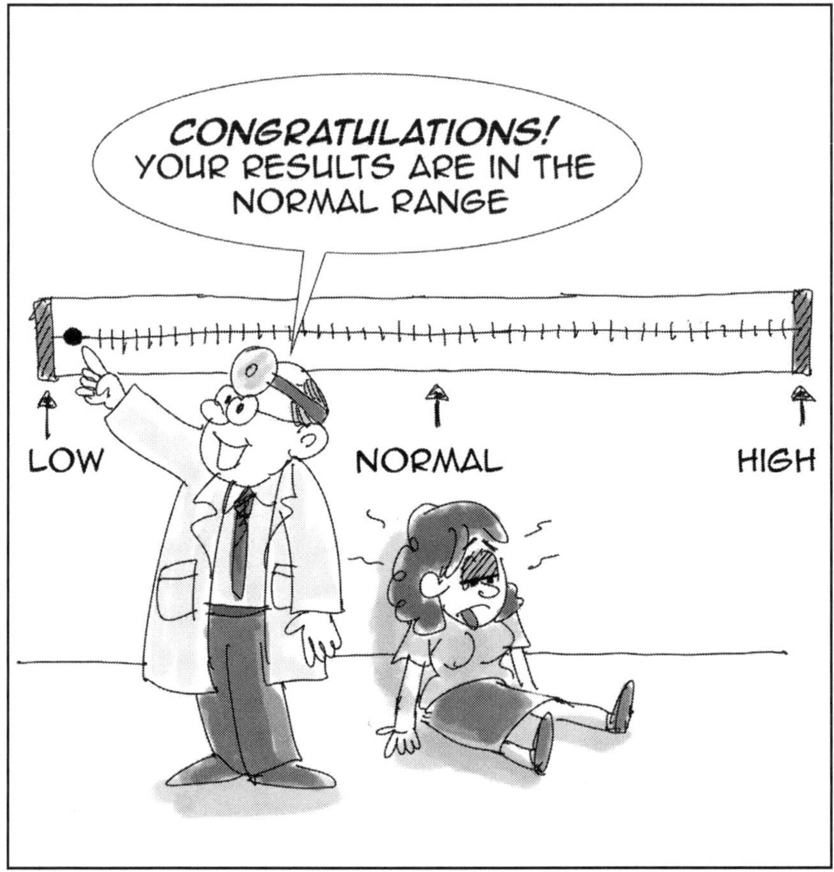

Another area in which to advocate for yourself is in the area of natural vitamin supplements. There is abundant scientific data supporting the use of these supplements, although not usually in the mainstream American medical journals. The problem, at least in the United States, is that doctors are generally not taught this information.

When my parents were in medical school in Argentina in the early 1960's, they received extended education in nutrition for several months. In the American medical school I attended in the 1980's, I had a nutrition class for the grand total of...one week. During this week we focused on details such as the illnesses that occur in the total absence of one vitamin (such as scurvy without vitamin C or beri-beri without vitamin B1). There was no mention of vitamins to support optimal health.

A wonderful ongoing study called the "90+ Study" has looked at supplement use and longevity.[20] Among their many findings in the people in this study, the use of supplements did not consistently correlate with living well into their nineties. The conventional medical world has used this information to say that supplements do not support optimal health and longevity. We will eventually learn how to tell who will and who won't benefit from vitamin supplements.

In particular, the emergence of genomics (the study of genetic alterations and how they affect your health) will help us identify who will and will not respond well to vitamins, supplements, and medications. For example, we know there is a gene that causes some people to make less vitamin D. They need to take higher doses of vitamin D supplementation to get a good blood level. For everyone, higher levels of this vitamin (which is actually a hormone[21]) are correlated with lower incidence of several cancers, heart disease, and osteoporosis. For people with the gene alteration, they need even higher doses to reap the benefits.

The dosing of vitamin D also gives us another example of the difference between conventional medicine and anti-aging/regenerative medicine. The recommended daily allowance (RDA) set by the Institute of Medicine for vitamin D is 800 iu (international units) per day. This rarely gives anyone an optimal blood level of vitamin D. Daily amounts of vitamin D can be as high as 5000 iu or more. There are rare reports of toxicity with vitamin D, but only in people taking over 300,000 iu per week. So, even if you have a doctor trying to keep up with current approaches such as optimizing vitamin D levels, you still need to advocate for yourself to make sure you are getting a high enough dose and getting your level tested.

GO FOR "OPTIMAL"

As we said, all too often when you go to the doctor and they order blood work on you, if your results come out barely inside the laboratory reference range, you will be told your results are normal. Whenever a patient tells me their results were normal, I always cringe just a little. I cringe because I know that doctors are eager to check the test off of their list and move on rather than look out for what is actually an optimal level for the patient.

Many, if not most doctors, base their clinical decisions on information given to them during their medical training. It takes a strong personal commitment for a doctor to stay up to date on the medical information that keeps emerging at an accelerating pace.

> A report from the Institute of Medicine found that it takes an average of 17 years from the publication of new scientific data to change how doctors actually practice medicine.[13]

The goal of practicing evidence-based medicine requires attending conferences, reading journals, and actively looking outside the box. It also calls for treating patients as whole individuals, which takes more time than only prescribing a medication to treat a symptom.

"NORMAL" VS. "OPTIMAL"

Let me use thyroid testing as an example to show you the difference between "normal" and "optimal." Most doctors check your thyroid level by measuring one test: the TSH test. Most labs have a reference range for this test that goes up to about 4.5. This is a case of a test where a higher level is not better.

I have patients whose level goes up to eight or nine and they are still told that the doctor is "just going to keep an eye on it" and recheck it in a few months. This is even though they are far outside the "normal range"! Even many people with a TSH level inside the "normal range" (up to 4.5) suffer from symptoms of low thyroid function, including fatigue, infertility, depression, mental fog, constipation, muscle weakness, or obesity.

In most people, an optimal TSH is actually at or just below 1.0. Also, there are many factors that makes a TSH level appear lower. For example, in someone who is overweight or obese, the fat tissue they are carrying is hormonally active and actually causes the TSH level to be lower, or closer to the "normal" range. This is so unfortunate because most people who struggle with their weight or have other symptoms of low thyroid function would benefit from support of their thyroid hormone system.

A bit of history on the TSH test:

Before the TSH lab test was put into wide use in the 1960's, people with symptoms of low thyroid function were simply treated with thyroid medication to see if their symptoms improved. At this point in time, the vast majority of doctors in the United States base treatment for thyroid symptoms entirely on the TSH test result rather than patient symptoms and response.

Let me also add that the TSH test is not the only way to measure thyroid hormone levels. TSH is Thyroid Stimulating Hormone, which the brain releases in order to stimulate the thyroid gland to make the inactive form of thyroid hormone

– thyroxine, or T4 – which then has to convert to the active form – triiodothyronine, or T3. Under physiologic stress, however, the T4, instead of being converted into the active T3 (in the liver, muscle and other tissues), can be converted into a blocking form of thyroid hormone – reverse T3.

I continue to be amazed by how many doctors, even endocrinologists, refuse to do these additional tests (free T4, free T3, reverse T3, anti-thyroid antibodies, iodine level) to get a more accurate picture of thyroid hormone levels in their patients. This information, by the way, is in the standard endocrinology literature, not just in alternative medical journals and web sites. We mentioned above the seventeen years (or more) delay in information going from publication to being used in clinical practice. Treatment of low thyroid is a classic case of this problem.

Another important example of "normal" vs. "optimal" is your vitamin D level. Most lab reference ranges go from thirty up to eighty. In other words, if your level is thirty-one, you will be told that your level is "normal" (again, that word that often makes me cringe).

An optimal level of vitamin D, however, is between 60 and 80 ng/ml, or higher if you are not feeling well or dealing with any kind of illness.

Earlier, we discussed that the RDA of vitamin D is 800 iu, which is not nearly enough to help you reach an optimal blood level of the active form of vitamin D (the test for the active form, by the way, is "25-OH-vitamin D").

Depending on the lab definition of "normal", up to seventy-five percent of people in the United States have a low vitamin D level and would benefit from supplementation.[22] A good daily dose of vitamin D is usually between 2,000 and 5,000 iu. Personally, I prefer the weekly dose of 50,000 iu for convenience (and taking fewer capsules during the week).

This works because vitamin D is fat-soluble and stores in the fat without building up to toxic levels. Like we said before, it is VERY difficult to overdose on vitamin D. It has many demonstrated health benefits, and I recommend that everyone supplement to get an optimal level of vitamin D.

DO STATISTICS APPLY TO YOU?

It is challenging to design a study that will show significant differences between study groups. Without getting into the details of study design (there are entire university departments dedicated to this), studies conducted in groups will yield results for the group, not each individual. The number of people in a study group is referred to as "n".

For example, if a drug causes vomiting in ten percent of people who take it, this is not the percentage that applies to you. For you it is either zero percent or one hundred percent. While it is valuable to know that ten percent of a group had that side effect, please remember that you are an individual. The percentage in the group is an indicator of what *might* happen to you. *You* are an "n of 1".

Last but not least, that "normal" range for your lab result? It is usually just a reporting by the lab of the range of results in the middle ninety-five percent of people who took that test. I have actually seen some lab ranges go down over time, as people have lower levels of various vitamins and hormones as we get less healthy as a society.

Do not just settle for being in the "normal range". The bottom line is that YOU must advocate for yourself with your doctor in order to sail past "normal" and get to "optimal" so you can go for GREAT.

We have arrived at the last step in our five-step formula.

Patient Name: You!

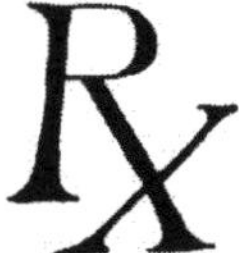

ADVOCATE FOR YOURSELF

Tips for Success:

- **Be the tail that wags the dog**
- **Reject the word "just"**
- **Go for *optimal***
- **Beware the "normal range"**
- **Get treated as the individual you are**

Signature: Dr. Liz, M.D.

CHAPTER 5
T IS FOR THRIVE

Welcome to Step 5!

DON'T JUST SURVIVE, GO FOR THRIVE

So, you have reached the Holy Grail. Balance. Feeling GREAT. Now what?

Do you roll the dice and pray it will last? Do you try to stay excited so you will stay on track?

Here is the deal with being human: enthusiasm fades. Therefore, you must be proactive about staying in balance and feeling your best.

New is exciting, but then daily routines and obligations set in and the "new" becomes the "old", or at least the "usual". This happens all the way down to our cells.

MAINTENANCE MINDSET

As celebrity nutritionist JJ Virgin says in her book *The Virgin Diet*, "There's an important behavior difference between dating and marriage."

One set of behaviors gets you to a goal. Another set of behaviors keeps you there.

Weight loss is a perfect example. If you have twenty-five pounds to lose, you have to make changes that increase your burn rate of the extra fuel your body is carrying. This includes changes in what and how much you eat, and how you move your body. How many programs are out there to help you do this? Too many to count.

In order to keep the weight off, though, you have to settle in for the long term. You do not go anymore to the areas of the supermarket that have the foods that got your weight up in the first place. Exercise has a new place in your weekly schedule that you make a top priority.

Once you achieve a goal, which in this case is feeling GREAT, you have to adjust your behaviors to maintain your new status of having balanced hormones. In fact, as we have said, it is not hormone balance, but rather *hormone balancing.*

Hormone balancing is an ongoing project for the rest of your life.

MAINTENANCE SUPPORT STRUCTURE

How will you adjust your daily routine to support the results that new hormone levels and new behaviors will give you?

In addition to too-many-to-count diet programs, there are too-many-to-count programs out there to help you stay on track. Here are some of my tips and suggestions to keep you on track and consistently stay proactive about feeling your best.

If you are at a starting point on your journey to feeling GREAT, and you feel overloaded with information, try this:

Pick ONE program that you like and stay with it in the long run. Or, pick features of various programs to fashion your own path. What matters is that you have some kind of path that helps YOU stay on track and feel your best.

Whatever program you pick, ask yourself: Does this program support me in all of the areas of being human and owning a human body?

- Nutrition
- Exercise
- Hormone balancing
- Spirit

When it comes to healthy eating, for example, I like to refer to the "human program", i.e. what our DNA is programmed for. I agree with the experts who observe that humans are omnivorous (eating both plants and animals for nourishment) based on the fact that we have sharp incising teeth in the front of our mouths (able to cut into flesh) and flat teeth in the back (able to grind plants).

Eggs are an interesting food item; they fall outside the "catch it or pick it" qualifying feature of lean proteins or plants. I did have one patient who vigorously disagreed with me, saying that of course humans are programmed to collect and eat eggs due to our fingers which nicely interlace to form a perfect basket shape to reach into a nest and gather eggs to eat. Many eating programs which focus on food intolerance (autoimmune issues with food) have people remove eggs from their diet. Removing food-intolerance foods often yields weight loss results in people who were previously stuck even though they were eating cleanly.

For health and longevity, and some say also for weight

loss, intermittent fasting has a big scientific and popular following. Because this information emerges and changes at such a rapid pace, I like to keep my patients and readers posted on latest information by posting it on my website. Please visit www.DrLizMD.com to make sure you are part of my online community to receive my latest updates and recommendations on trends such as intermittent fasting.

CHECK-IN PLAN

Even though you brush your teeth regularly, I also assume that you go to the dentist on a somewhat regular basis, right?

Even though you can read about how to accomplish good oral health (which by the way is very important to avoid cardiovascular disease, the number one killer in the United States) you still need some external verification that you are doing a good job and that your body is not developing issues that are not producing symptoms yet.

To support you on your lifetime journey of feeling GREAT you need to assemble your own team of practitioners who listen to you and respond to changing circumstances and needs in your life. Depending on how many health issues you have, you may need a bigger team. You do always need, though, a primary doctor – someone who listens to you and responds to your needs.

It is a tough time for patients and for doctors right now. I think the only people benefitting from the current health insurance system in the United States are the CEO's of the insurance companies.

Hopefully you have medical insurance. Even though your primary doctor on your insurance does not have much time to spend with you each time you go in, you can take steps to be ready to make the most of her or his time. Please see the Resources section for a link to a checklist to use before an appointment with your doctor, to make sure you get questions answered and your medical needs met.

Unfortunately, the current American medical system divides up the human body into its organs and organ systems instead of considering how they work together. **Functional medicine** refers to an approach focused on the good functioning of the organs and systems in the human body. Instead of looking at one organ in isolation, doctors who practice functional medicine look at the body as a whole (also called a holistic approach).

Again, because so many doctors who accept medical insurance are so strapped for time, they will often take a symptom and connect it to one particular organ malfunction or illness in order to give a drug to alleviate the symptom. They do have the goal of helping you feel better by clearing up the symptom, but this usually ends up being a "Band-Aid®" approach instead of a holistic approach.

"Functional medicine" is distinct from but related to "integrative medicine." A definition that I like for integrative medicine is from the government agency, the National Center for Complementary and Alternative Medicine:

> "Integrative health care often brings conventional and complementary approaches together in a coordinated way. It emphasizes a holistic, patient-focused approach to health care and wellness—often including mental, emotional, functional, spiritual, social, and community aspects—and treating the whole person rather than, for example, one organ system. It aims for well-coordinated care between different providers and institutions."[23]

Even if your doctor does not call him or herself an Integrative Medicine doctor, you can still tell if your symptoms are being treated with "Band-Aids®", or if your doctor is looking at you as a whole person and trying their best to find out underlying causes of what is going on.

DON'T CATCH "LABELITIS"

A caution about diagnoses and diagnosis codes: these codes are usually the bane of a doctor's existence, and are make-or-break for insurance companies to pay for the services you are using. While you do not need to learn diagnosis codes, you do want to understand that using them attaches the diagnosis label to you in the insurance realm, probably forever. This can work for you in that it can increase the chances that your insurance will cover testing and treatments attached to a particular diagnosis. These labels can work against you in the insurance setting of "pre-existing conditions." The rules governing how insurance companies cover pre-existing conditions are, at the time of this writing, in favor of patients, but this is subject to political change.

That said, I really do not like labels. YOU are the person who is **currently** experiencing a certain symptom.

Do not identify with a diagnosis, as in saying "I **AM** a diabetic." Instead, say "I **have** diabetes" as a way to say that your body is currently facing a challenge processing sugar, and that you are able to influence this process with your choices of lifestyle and medical care, including regular and complementary interventions.

How will you find the best people for your health success team?

You have many choices: medical doctors, nurse practitioners, physician assistants, nutritionists, health coaches, chiropractors, acupuncturists, and so on. You will decide who is an appropriate member of your team. I encourage you to choose each member of this team to be someone who contributes to your experience of being supported on your journey (including your interactions with their staff).

PERSONALIZE YOUR PLAN

Part of feeling supported is experiencing a personal connection.

Luckily, this does not require a lot of personal time spent with you, although of course that is nice. Again, not every doctor, especially doctors who bill insurance, can spend the kind of time with you that a doctor who does not bill insurance might be able to.[24]

You can feel a personal connection with an expert you have met only briefly, or even have never met. You can resonate with what they express, write about or speak about.

For example, I feel very personally connected with the work of Dr. Christiane Northrup. She has written so many bestselling books about women's health and menopause that it shocks me when I meet someone who has not heard of her. I have met her on at least two occasions when I have heard her speak at events, always of course getting a picture with her! I was blessed to have her endorse my first book, "Dr. Liz's Easy Guide to Menopause".

Dr. Northrup is an example of an expert who is *my* leading edge, encouraging me to continue learning and looking at my own life for areas to improve and expand. She is one of my gurus.

In addition to Dr. Christiane Northrup, other gurus I follow include:

- Dr. Sara Gottfried – especially her writing on the impact of genes on our health, and the brain-gut connection
- Nutritionist JJ Virgin – almost every day I refer patients to her work on removing food-intolerance foods from their diets
- Entrepreneur and coach extraordinaire Lisa Sasevich – for her business leadership
- Bobbi Palmer, Dating Coach for Women Over 40 – I am a student of hers and I refer people to her work all the time
- And a handful of others – Oprah, Suzanne Somers, and other inspiring people.

The word "guru" has its origin in the Sanskrit for "elder" or "teacher". Its Latin word connection is to "gravis", meaning "heavy, or weighty" as in "venerable, worthy of honor."

WHO ARE *YOUR* GURUS?

While the internet has helped both worthy and not-so-worthy gurus obtain a big following online, my point still stands that you can find a person or handful of people whose words, videos, and messages resonate with you, and encourage and support you on your journey.

They are people who honor you and your goals for your health and your life.

In fact, the variety of people and ideas available online can support you in including some variety of ideas and methods to keep you inspired and engaged with your own learning and growing, to stay in your best health.

Humans are programmed to seek some variety in our

lives. Make sure your plan to maintain the balance and feeling great that you have worked so hard to achieve includes people and ideas that stimulate you, support you, and adapt with you to the changes you experience as life moves along.

Patient Name: You!

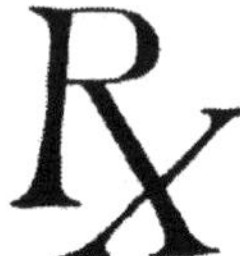

THRIVE

Tips for Success:

- **Develop a maintenance mindset**
- **Put in place a maintenance support structure**
- **Have a check-in plan with your health team**
- **Personalize your plan**
- **Pick a few favorite gurus to learn with and follow**

Signature: Dr. Liz, M.D.

CHAPTER 6

GREAT: WHERE DO WE GO FROM HERE?

> Karen came to me at age fifty-two. A professional woman with a rewarding career, grown kids, and a fulfilling intimate relationship, she wanted to address her perimenopausal symptoms that were not terrible, but still making her feel "off." Mild hot flashes and sleep disruption were lowering her energy level and giving her some headaches. We started her at first with some testosterone, adding some progesterone later, and finally a low dose of estrogen (all bioidentical, of course). Most recently, she has been enjoying her work, her relationship, her exciting travel, and her family. She is feeling GREAT.

My work with Karen provides a great illustration of my five-step formula for thriving at every age.

Step 1. Gain knowledge: Karen was aware of the changes in her body as she was getting older. She was willing to learn about bioidentical hormones and how to replenish them safely.

Step 2. Realize the truth about hormones: Karen was happy to learn that every scary thing she had heard about hormone replenishment was due to misinformation or misinterpretation of the data.

Step 3. Explore expectations: Karen managed her own expectations by also addressing her own nutrition, exercise, and spirit. She continues to do her part in our wonderful doctor-patient partnership.

Step 4. Advocate for yourself: Karen advocated for herself by going outside her insurance network to get the help she needed to feel her best. She is willing to be the tail that wags the dog.

Step 5. Thrive: In her relationships and her life, she is not willing to settle for just surviving – she wants to thrive, now and for the rest of her life!

FEEL GOOD AND DO GOOD

According to Dr. Pat Allen, women need to FEEL good in order to DO good, while men need to DO good in order to FEEL good.

Let's look at this for a moment.

If women need to feel good in order to do good, what happens when their hormones – the chemistry of our emotions – are out of whack? The phrase women use with me time and again is, "I just don't feel like myself."

Ladies, now you know you can safely use the right kinds of hormone replenishment to "feel like yourself again."

If men need to do good in order to feel good, what happens when hormone decline with age leaves them without the drive and ability to do their best?

Now you know that men can also safely use the right kinds of hormone replenishment to get back in gear.

Being "hormonal" is no fun for anyone. It affects the woman herself, and her partner, as well as anyone else in her close circle of friends, family or co-workers.

I see women running into hormonal hot water at younger and younger ages. This is due to what are called "endocrine disruptors", which are found in high amounts of sugar and fat in our diet, chemicals in processed foods, soaps and lotions, hormones in animal sources of food, and toxic chemicals in other products we use every day.

The good news is that our bodies are designed to detoxify our environment. Our part is to lower the toxic burden as much as possible. Having optimal hormone levels helps our cells function at their best capacity, including the cells of our organs that detoxify.

Balanced hormones help our metabolism work at its best. When we carry excess fat, that fat tissue does not just sit there bothering us, but it is actually hormonally working against us. Disrupted hormone levels contribute to slower metabolism.

Of course, we still have to pay attention to other factors in metabolism, including what we eat, how regularly we move our bodies, and how our gut is working. It is also critical to support our emotional and spiritual health.

Hormonal disruption and perimenopause are happening at younger ages also due to physiologic stress. Even though we are good at adapting to stressors in life, our cellular physiology may not adapt as easily to life as we now live it.

We live with certain constants that many of us have become used to, such as constant email, constant availability via cell phone, constant traffic.

I want women and men to feel their best AND do their best, not just for the world, but also for each other in their intimate relationships. I want people to invest in their hormone health so they do not end up paying even more to a divorce attorney later in life.

No one gets married thinking they will divorce, but if sex and sexuality leave a marriage against the wishes of one or both partners, the relationship will suffer.

I speak with women all the time about decreased libido, which I like to point out is not only about sex. Less desire for sex is usually accompanied by less motivation and drive in general. Lower *life energy.*

Fixing low libido is good for your health in general.

I know for men it is difficult if not impossible to bring up the issue of hormonal imbalance with the women in their lives. No one likes to be told she is "being hormonal"!

Women definitely do not like to be told they are hormonal; in fact, that can really be like sticking your hand in a blender. Men might not react as badly to being told they might have low hormone levels, but men do have a reputation for being reluctant to go to a doctor to get checked out.

When I started dating my husband, he was excited about the work I do and wanted me to check out his hormone levels. He had been working on weight loss for the year before we met, and he had already lost over sixty pounds. He felt pretty good but wanted to go for "optimal" – my kind of guy! His thyroid, adrenals, and vitamin levels were great; no wonder his efforts were working.

Getting to know each other, discovering intimacy in a grown-up way, blending our families (I got a wonderful bonus daughter and grand-daughter in our marriage), dealing with health challenges, and supporting each other in our work, have all been the gifts of our relationship. Working on my own hormone balancing, and supporting him in working on his is a journey we are committed to sharing for as many decades to come as possible.

Optimal health includes how we feel emotionally and the health of our relationships.

Just because hormone levels in women decrease with age, this does not mean that women need to be afraid of ways to replenish these hormones enough to feel good and enjoy the people in her life. Just because levels of testosterone decrease in men with age, this does not mean that men are destined to be the proverbial "boiling frog", who does not notice the water slowly warming to the point of danger.

I hope you have found this book helpful. I also hope you have a renewed motivation to reach and keep your best level of health, both for yourself and for the people in your life you care about the most.

If you are not already a part of my online community, please go to www.DrLizMD.com to receive my special reports on latest medical information to feel your best at every age.

I hope I have alleviated fears about using the right kinds of hormone replenishment to support you in feeling your best.

After reading this book, I hope you feel empowered to continually work to achieve and maintain good hormone balancing. Yes, hormone replenishment can sometimes lead to side effects, but I hope a little bit of facial hair or acne will not be enough to keep you from pursuing a level of hormone balance that will keep happiness and connection in your relationships.

Join me in going for the most vibrant health possible, for as long as possible. It is not about staying young forever. What good is extending our "lifespan" if we don't lengthen our "health span"?

I wish you a life of love, passion, and connection with those you care about. I wish you a long "health span" – a life of thinking your best thoughts, feeling your best feelings, and doing your best in all of your endeavors.

I hope I have motivated you to use this GREAT five-step formula so you can thrive at every age. Remember, getting older is a privilege, feeling old is optional.

Don't settle. Go for GREAT.

APPENDIX A – REFERENCES

CHAPTER 1

1. Gawande, Atul. Being Mortal, Picador/Metropolitan Books, New York, 2014.

2. Morgentaler, Abraham. Testosterone for Life: Recharge Your Vitality, Sex Drive, Muscle Mass, and Overall Health! McGraw-Hill Education, 2008.

3. Odds of getting hit by a car: https://www.reference.com/math/odds-getting-hit-car-8153e02f5ac36140

4. Risk of blood clot with oral contraceptive pill: https://www.acog.org/-/media/Committee-Opinions/Committee-on-Gynecologic-Practice/co540.pdf?dmc=1&ts=20190623T0423592424

5. Baseline incidence of blood clots in women ages 40 to 59: http://www.cheo.on.ca/uploads/genetics/Requisitions/Factor%20V%20English.pdf

6. Women's Health Initiative Study https://www.whi.org

CHAPTER 2

7. Postmenopausal Estrogen Therapy: Route of Administration and Risk of Venous Thromboembolism:

https://www.acog.org/-/media/Committee-Opinions/Committee-on-Gynecologic-Practice/co556.pdf?dmc=1&ts=20190623T0442170258

8. Bioidentical progesterone compared to progestin: https://www.ncbi.nlm.nih.gov/pubmed/19179815

9. Morgentaler, Abraham. Testosterone for Life: Recharge Your Vitality, Sex Drive, Muscle Mass, and Overall Health! McGraw-Hill Education, 2008.

10. Meta-analysis of the effect of testosterone treatment on prostate cancer: https://www.medscape.com/viewarticle/844907#vp_1

11. ACOG Practice Bulletin No. 141: Management of Menopausal Symptoms https://journals.lww.com/greenjournal/Abstract/2014/01000/Practice_Bulletin_No__141___Management_of.37.aspx

12. North American Menopause Society hormone therapy position statement: https://www.menopause.org/docs/default-source/2017/nams-2017-hormone-therapy-position-statement.pdf

13. Seventeen-year delay in new knowledge reaching doctors' practice: https://journals.sagepub.com/doi/abs/10.1177/152715440325830 4 and https://www.holtorfmed.com/download/doctors-knowledge/Why_Doesnt_My_Doctor_Know_This.pdf

14. Study showing doctors did better than a computer algorithm: https://www.forbes.com/sites/robertglatter/2016/10/13/doctors-beat-online-symptom-checkers-new-study-finds/#3245fcf52d44

CHAPTER 3

15. Lipton, Bruce, PhD. The Biology of Belief, Hay House, 2016.

16. https://www.drnorthrup.com/category/health/

17. https://www.ted.com/talks/jane_fonda_life_s_third_act?language=en

18. http://www.drlizmd.com/is-your-brain-on-fire/

19. Plate size: https://www.parentingnh.com/size-really-does-matter/

CHAPTER 4

20. 90+ Study: http://www.mind.uci.edu/research-studies/90plus-study/

21. Vitamin D is actually a hormone: http://www.drlizmd.com/vitamin-d-sunshine-hormone/

22. https://www.scientificamerican.com/article/vitamin-d-deficiency-united-states/

CHAPTER 5

23. Definition of integrative health: https://nccih.nih.gov/health/integrative-health

24. http://www.drlizmd.com/dont-take-insurance/

APPENDIX B – RESOURCES

FOR LINKS, GO TO HTTP://WWW.DRLIZMD.COM/ BOOKRESOURCES

Dr. Susan Peirce Thompson, PhD

- Bright Line Eating is the most scientifically-based eating program for weight loss and healing food addiction that I have ever learned about (and that is saying something, since patients have been introducing me to weight loss programs and fads for the past 30 years). I enjoy her videos and online support materials. Also, my husband and I have been losing weight comfortably on her program.

Alison Armstrong

- I have personally known Alison Armstrong since 1986. The creator of the Queen's Code series of courses and books, Alison's work has been essential to my understanding of men, women, and all the types of relationships we engage in, including at work and at home with children. I have taken most of her courses; I find her work to be transformational.

Dr. Christiane Northrup, MD

- Dr. Chris is the leading thinker of our time about the spiritual aspect of health and how important our mindset is to our success (in health and every other area of our lives). I first met Dr. Chris in 2009, having followed her already for some time. Since then, I go to hear her speak as often as possible, and I enjoy the resources she provides online.

Suzanne Somers

- You know her as a famous television actress, but did you know she has written **twenty-five** books and counting? Suzanne is also an amazing speaker! She is the best celebrity advocate of bioidentical hormone therapy on the planet, as far as I am concerned.

Haylie Pomroy

- Fast Metabolism Diet is an eating program that approaches the body the way I do, addressing what foods and exercise methods stimulate the thyroid gland, the adrenal glands, and so on. Haylie's program rotates food and exercise during the week, validating what I have been saying to patients for years about how to keep your metabolism going strong.

Dr. Sara Gottfried

- A fellow Bay area resident (and also fellow former OB/GYN doctor), Sara Gottfried is on the cutting edge of incorporating genomics into our understanding of health care. She shares my passion for aging with strength and grace.

Dr. Pat Allen

- Dr. Pat is in her 80's and going strong! She was on Oprah many times; if you haven't heard of her, it's because Oprah didn't like her direct "tell it like it is" style. In her books on dating and marriage, her no-nonsense approach to masculine and feminine energy has changed my relationships and my life.

JJ Virgin

- JJ's approach to eating and weight loss focuses on (1) removing foods that many people are intolerant of, and (2) removing sources of hidden sugar. Her work is essential to dealing with the food sensitivities women deal with as we get older and our hormones go out of balance (not to mention her recipes!).

Landmark Education

- After first participating in this curriculum of personal development and transformational programs at the age of 19, I include myself in the 94% of people surveyed who have done these courses who say it made a profound and lasting difference in their lives. It is not therapeutic in nature, and therefore not right for every person or every situation. However, I will say that the people closest to me in my life have done these courses, giving us a deep bond in life.

Steven Campbell, M.S.

- Steven is "the brain whisperer." His book, Making Your Brain Magnificent, is the best summary I have seen of brain science over the last few decades to help you become friends with your thoughts so that you can have love yourself powerfully. Every chapter of his book and the classes he teaches give practical tips and tools to apply this knowledge, and help you make your dreams come true. Steven says, "Decades of studies on emotional well-being have proven one important fact: contentment is within the control of every one of us."

Bobbi Palmer

- I recommend all women over 40 (and sometimes even younger) get to know Bobbi's information on dating and relationships in midlife and beyond. Bobbi met and married her husband at the age of 47. She combines her own story with deep knowledge and expertise on relationships between men and women, providing humorous and wise articles and videos. My work with Bobbi helped me achieve my own "grown-up love story."

ABOUT THE AUTHOR

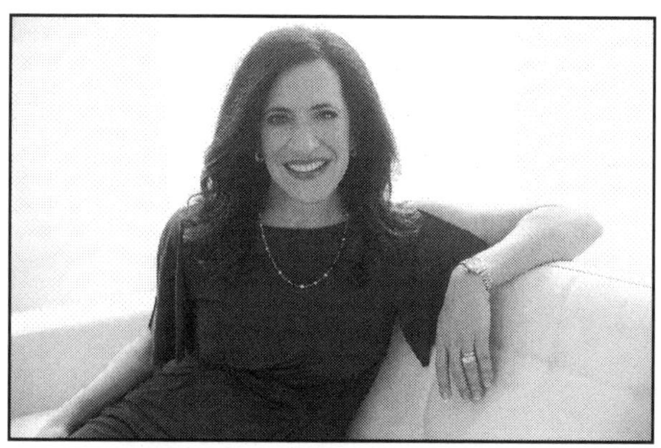

As a doctor for almost 30 years, Dr. Liz Lyster has helped women and men regain energy, reignite their sex drive, clear up hormonal imbalance, and lose hundreds of pounds. After graduating from Cornell University with honors, she went to medical school at the University of California, Irvine, then did her OB/GYN residency in Los Angeles. To expand her commitment to teaching, Dr. Liz achieved a Masters of Public Health degree from UCLA in Community Health Education. Dr. Liz currently teaches part-time at Notre Dame de Namur University in Belmont, California, in addition to her private medical practice in Foster City, CA.

Dr. Liz practices what she preaches. To model growing older with grace, agility and power, Dr. Liz celebrated turning fifty by climbing Mt. Kilimanjaro. She is the mom of two young adult sons, and enjoys traveling, hiking and Argentine tango dancing with her husband.

Dr. Liz writes and speaks as often as possible. She would be delighted to welcome you to her online community, speak for your group, or consult with you in person in her practice. She can be reached via her web site at www.DrLizMD.com.

TAKE NOTES & WRITE DOWN YOUR NEXT STEPS TO GO FOR GREAT!

Made in the USA
Columbia, SC
01 October 2024